# Smoothies for Weight Loss, Health, and Beauty

*Healthy, Delicious, Quick, and Easy Smoothie Recipe Book for Beginners*

**Holly Johnson**

# Table of Contents

# Introduction

Too many people today suffer from severe health problems that cause weight gain, dull skin, weak and thin hair, and low energy. The rigors of daily life make it difficult to plan out healthy, low-calorie meals that will make you feel better. Most of the time, people with these problems simply wish them away, never knowing how to truly fix them.

Luckily, there is an entire genre of foods that you can make in under five minutes that will give you the nutrition you need: smoothies. Green smoothies give you the nutrients necessary to make it through a long day. Waking up with protein shakes will make you feel more energized and, consequently, will encourage you to be more active. Fruit and vegetable smoothies give you the requirements most people don't get in a day. The ingredients in smoothies are both delicious and incredibly healthy.

My name is Holly Johnson, and I'm a nutritionist. I'm a mother of two children and an enthusiast for healthy lifestyles. I love to cook and am constantly looking for new, interesting recipes. I prefer healthy foods rich in nutrients to make me and others feel full of energy all day long. I'm also an exercise enthusiast that enjoys long walks and practicing yoga. It's my goal to make you feel strong and healthy in your life.

When you read this book, you'll receive insight on which ingredients will improve your health and how to create your own smoothies that are both healthy and delicious. These smoothies give you the head start you need in the morning, for snacks, and after workouts. When you start eating these smoothies daily, you'll see your life change for the better.

Smoothies are beneficial for weight loss and healthy living, so when you follow these recipes, you make a promise to yourself to improve. Thousands of individuals have seen results from eating smoothies daily, and you can, too. If you're experiencing dull skin, weak and thin hair, weight gain, lack of energy, or a host of other possible problems, this book can help you find solutions.

Millions of people suffer needlessly with problems they can either fix or seriously improve, so don't wait around. It's important to investigate and find a solution for your health problems before they get too severe. Your health should be a top priority.

If you're ready to start thinking about yourself and improve your life, there's never a better time to start. The more time you spend on yourself, the more time you'll have for others. Too few people recognize the importance of self-health. Don't be a part of that silent majority and take your health into your own hands today.

# Chapter 1: The Benefits of Smoothies

Years of crazy dieting have probably taught you to count calories and actively seek foods that are low in carbohydrates and high in protein. However, finding the right balance of nutrients is often difficult if you don't know what you're doing. Dieting can cause a lack of energy and even cause stress.

So, before you start down that frustrating road again, consider investing in foods that will taste delicious and give you that energy boost you're always craving. Smoothies come in a wide variety of flavors and can give you an incredible nutritional advantage. After all, who doesn't want a delicious boost that will keep them coming back for more?

## Smoothies and Weight Loss

You've no doubt heard of meal replacement shakes and smoothies that theoretically can cure any ill, but there is no scientific backing for these pre-packaged smoothies. These beverages are usually loaded with sugar, and you don't always know what you're getting unless you consult a nutritionist. In fact, a study conducted by Kimberly A. Gudzune et al. (2015) analyzed 45 studies regarding these commercial products and found that most are not only unhelpful, but may ultimately slow your weight loss in the future if you don't pair them with exercise.

Sugary foods and drinks are one of the leading causes of weight gain, but not for the reason you may think. True, they are typically packed with calories, but sugary products are also responsible for your cravings. The more sugar you consume, the more likely you are to go back for more. Commercial smoothies and meal replacement shakes capitalize on this and encourage you to always come back for more.

Homemade smoothies are much better for you and are often cheaper and faster to make as well. You can control your sugar intake and blend in additives that will improve your health. They are also an excellent replacement for unhealthy eating: most people use them as a substitute for eating fried foods and snacks loaded with sugar.

The vitamins and minerals found in smoothies can fill you up while maintaining your body's ability to burn fat. Once filled up, you won't be as tempted to eat. Eating too much or too little is typically the cause of weight gain, but eating fresh fruits and vegetables gives your body the nutrition it needs while sustaining you until your next meal.

How long it takes to consume a meal also plays a large part in how much you will consume. Consuming a smoothie quickly will likely leave you wanting more a short time later. However, if you consume it slowly, taking spoonfuls at a time instead of large gulps, you'll find yourself fuller for longer. Because smoothies are blended fruits and vegetables, it's easier and quicker to consume them, which is why most dieticians prefer to eat whole fruits and vegetables. However, smoothies that are eaten slower often have the same staying power that whole fruits and vegetables do.

In a study conducted by Peter J. Rogers and Roya Shahrokni (2018), 48 healthy adults tested the effectiveness of fruit smoothies in keeping participants full in comparison to sugary fruit drinks and a fruit cocktail. They discovered that two minutes after consuming the products, smoothies were more likely than both sugary drinks and the fruit cocktails to keep participants full. After two hours, smoothies were again at the top of the list.

Of course, the best way to effectively lose weight eating smoothies is to combine their consumption with consistent exercise. Any dietary change requires exercise to reach peak effectiveness. Smoothies will likely make you feel more energetic, so use the energy wisely.

## Smoothies and Health

Most people who start drinking smoothies recognize a difference in their lives shortly after starting. Why? Most people don't incorporate enough vitamins and minerals in their diets that are often found in fruits and vegetables.

Fruit smoothies are primarily eaten for breakfast because their high carbohydrate rate can ensure that you'll have enough energy for the rest of the day. Also, consuming large amounts of carbohydrates in the morning gives your body the chance to use them instead of putting them into storage in the form of fat. However, if you include a smattering of protein and vegetable additives, it's possible to eat them throughout the day.

Green smoothies are a great option for people who struggle to stomach vegetables. Green smoothies typically include leafy greens that can still taste like the raspberry peach smoothie you were hoping for. They are also a great source of fiber and vitamins A and K. The key is to add ingredients that will ultimately help you become healthier while letting you enjoy a great taste.

## Mistakes and Fixes for Smoothies

Many people throw in as many fruits and vegetables as they can into a smoothie, hoping that the more they add, the healthier it will be. However, this common mistake often leads people into more problems. Here are some of the most common mistakes and how to fix them.

### Smoothie Glass is Too Large

Popular smoothie destinations are thriving because they give people what they want: a feeling of health when consuming a 24 oz tub of smoothie. The problem is that most people would never consume that many raw fruits and vegetables. The thought of consuming a 24 oz container of strawberries is often enough to make even the healthiest person turn tail and run.

When making your smoothies, opt for 8-10 oz and save the rest. You typically don't need the extra granola or fruits that come with commercial smoothies. Spread out your smoothie intake to two days if you get such a large smoothie. You should only consume one small smoothie per day for either breakfast, lunch, or dinner.

### Smoothie Ingredient Overload

Another common mistake is overloading smoothies with many unnecessary ingredients. Even though most fruit and vegetables are fairly low in calories, adding a wide variety of ingredients adds up quickly. Forego whipped cream or ice cream, which often doubles or even triples the number of calories. Smoothies should be a quick snack and not an event.

If you're concerned about how many ingredients you're adding, keep a log of what you put into your blender. Check for the caloric amount and keep an eye on the benefits you're getting from the smoothie. Add ingredients such as coconut oil or avocado to give you extra flavor and creaminess without overloading you with calories.

### Too Many Sweeteners

Check the smoothies at grocery stores or famous smoothie places to see how much sugar is packed into popular items. You'll probably be surprised to see that most large smoothies contain more than 20 grams of sugar. Additives like honey or syrup can make you feel drowsy and easily irritated after several swigs, and your blood sugar will most likely go through the roof.

Luckily, you're well on your way to fixing this mistake by reading this book! Making your own smoothies is the key to remove the excess sugar you'd find in other commercial smoothies. Keep an eye on what you're adding to the smoothie and include low-calorie greens to keep the sugar content down.

*Slurping Your Smoothie*

Because smoothies are generally made to easily slide down your gullet, many people opt to consume thin smoothies similarly to how they would consume a beverage. However, eating quickly can cause you to gain weight and not get the most out of your smoothie. In a few hours, you'll start to feel major hunger pangs.

To fix the issue, eat smoothies with a spoon. Not only will this force you to slow down, but it will also make you thicken up your smoothies by adding yogurt or protein powders. Eating with a spoon also means that you can add products that are full of fiber, like chia seeds or flax meal.


**Improving Your Daily Intake**


Smoothies are remarkably helpful in diversifying your daily caloric intake. Fruits and vegetables contain fiber, antioxidants, vitamins, and minerals that you can't find in most other foods, especially snacks or quick meals (Hill, 2020). A balanced diet can reduce inflammation in injuries and prevent diseases such as heart disease or diabetes. Fruits and vegetables included in diets can also stave off osteoporosis and may prevent mental health decline.

Smoothies are usually a good source of fiber, which is also proven to reduce a wide variety of illnesses. Most people don't receive enough daily fiber, which leaves many sluggish and with the inability to focus. Western diets are typically not conducive to high fiber diets.

The World Health Organization (WHO) advocates for the food pyramid because it gives you a more balanced diet than most people receive. Adding a smoothie to your daily routine can often compensate for nutrients lost during a busy schedule. Fast food and dependence on high-carb diets make most people forget about the dietary benefits of fruits and vegetables, but smoothies are a quick fix if you have the right ingredients.

# Smoothies and Beauty

Everyone wants to experience a happy gut, but smoothies have another benefit as well: glowing skin. The nutrients you find in smoothies are responsible for your skin feeling and looking amazing. Of course, varying types of smoothies have varying types of results. For example, blackberries are rich in zinc, a mineral responsible for clearing up acne. Any variation in your diet can reveal vast changes in your skin.

### *Why Build Healthy Skin and How Smoothies Can Help*

If you were asked what the largest organ in the body was, you may turn to the small intestine or liver, but skin ultimately takes the cake. The skin needs to be protected from both external interactions and food consumption. UV light can cause skin cancer, but eating greasy foods constantly will also show brightly on your skin. The oils produced from your consumption of fat—and subsequent acne that appears—show more than any suntan.

If you've ever consumed prepackaged vitamins, you've likely felt disappointed with the results. Unfortunately, the truth is that most commercial vitamins don't help as much as regular consumption of the vitamins and minerals in food. Fruits and vegetables, some of the ultimate sources of vitamin and mineral deposits, give you the nutrients you need in a way that your body can digest well.

In a study conducted by Kok Wei Tan et al. (2015), fruit and vegetable smoothies were tested to find whether carotenoids helped skin improve. Carotenoids are red, yellow, and orange pigments typically found in fruits and vegetables and are potentially healthy to human skin. Eighty-one Malaysians participated in the experiment with one group consuming fruit and vegetable smoothies while the others drank only mineral water.

Those that consumed the smoothies showed a marked increase in redness and yellowness of the skin with a lower luminesce than the control group. Tan et al. (2015) suggested that the increase in color is possibly a result of extra blood flowing to the face, resulting in a healthier glow. The increase of color in the face is also commonly associated with physical attractiveness because of this healthy appearance.

***Nutrients Needed in a Smoothie***

The skin is the body's first barrier to external attacks. As such, the skin must have essential vitamins and minerals to increase its strength. You can generally see how healthy a person is by the way they look. Unnaturally pale people often have vitamin and mineral deficiencies. People with highly dull or glossy skin also appear sickly.

The most common vitamins and minerals that keep the body looking healthy are collagen, iron, coenzyme Q10, zinc, selenium, astaxanthin, vitamins C and E, folic acid, vitamins A and D, omega fatty acids, and β-carotene (McKeown, 2020). These vitamins not only prevent blemishes but can also fight against burns and the effects of harmful UV rays.

Folic acid is commonly associated with pregnancy health due to its role in healthy brain growth. However, folic acid is also responsible for making skin glow by sending oxygen-enriched blood to the surface. Folic acid is abundant in many vegetables including spinach and leafy greens, but it's also available in citrus fruits.

The benefits of vitamin A cannot be understated. It is often associated with immune system improvement. Enough vitamin A on the skin can successfully repel pathogens that are present on the surface of the skin due to microbes. Vitamin A is commonly introduced to patients who have an infection due to bacterial growth at the surface of the skin. Carrots, apricots, leafy greens, and sweet potatoes are all excellent sources of vitamin A. If you're feeling adventurous, also consider adding red pepper or cayenne to your smoothie.

Vitamin C is, perhaps, one of the best vitamins to add to your smoothie. Before the 1800s, sailors often picked up scurvy, the terrible disease that caused the swelling of gums and reopening of old wounds. The cure was extraordinarily simple, but it still plagues people today. Add vitamin C to your diet by including lemons, limes, oranges, or any other members of the citrus family to stave off scurvy effects.

Omega-3 and omega-6 fatty acids are responsible for keeping the body properly supplied with natural oils. People who are omega-3 or omega-6 deficient usually have dry skin, while those overindulging in fatty foods may experience acne. Consult a nutritionist or physician if you believe you're overeating foods containing these acids. Hemp seeds, walnuts, and chia seeds generally have omega-3 fatty acids while peanut butter and sunflower seeds are good sources of omega-6.

# Chapter 2: How to Make Smoothies

Though hardly the most overwhelming meal to make, smoothies require their own adjustments to make them creamy and delicious. Most of the time, you'll have to experiment with the recipes to make them work for you. Smoothies must also be the right consistency to get the most out of them. So, before you dive into making your smoothie, note these steps to creating the perfect smoothie.

## Step 1: Choose the Fruits and Vegetables

Picking the right fruit for a smoothie can seem like a chore, but it doesn't have to be. The key is to find fruits and vegetables with the vitamins and minerals you want and add them in the right proportions. Remember, you shouldn't consume more than 8-10 oz of smoothie per day. One cup is equal to 8 fluid oz, so if you're planning on splitting the number of fruits and vegetables in your smoothie, plan accordingly.

### *Start Fresh*

If choosing fresh fruit, calculate when you'll need to make the smoothies. For example, if you buy produce for a week, keep in mind that an avocado that is ripe on day one will not be ripe on day seven. There are methods to picking fruits and vegetables with longer shelf lives that will ultimately save you time and money.

Leafy greens tell you a lot about their condition based on their outside appearance. For instance, leafy greens showing any yellowing or soft spots are likely past their prime. Also, look out for the weight of your vegetables: They should feel heavy and full of moisture.

### *Containers*

Where you place your produce also plays a large role in how long they'll be ripe, so don't rush to the refrigerator after every purchase. The three main factors for a fruit or vegetable's shelf life are temperature, airflow, and the chemical excrement of plants, typically ethylene. Pay attention to where the fruits and vegetables grow. For instance, root vegetables are typically most at home in cool, dark areas.

Many fruits release ethylene on their own that forces them to age quicker. Leafy greens are especially susceptible to ethylene, and they will decay faster when they are stored next to fruits like apples and bananas. The reason for the separate containers for fruits and vegetables in the refrigerator is to keep your produce fresh for as long as possible.

Produce that is commonly left out typically needs more room to breathe. Your fruits and vegetables stored at room temperature will start to disintegrate faster when stored in a sealed container. Bananas and apples are other examples of this: the longer they're in a bag, even a perforated bag, the faster they'll ripen. On the flip side, produce that requires refrigeration typically requires sealing. These fruits and vegetables need moisture to maintain freshness. Typically, these types of fruits and vegetables are also more sensitive to ethylene, so sealing them provides an extra layer of protection.

If you're unsure about which fruits and vegetables to put where, conduct a google search. Most resources have a set plan for purchase and can help you decide what to buy at what times. When in doubt, experiment on your own. Find out how long fruits and vegetables can last by setting up a schedule and following your results. In many cases, the information you receive will be more beneficial to you than searching online since the change in humidity, temperature, and elevation are unique for every location.


***Fresh Vs Frozen***


Frozen fruits and vegetables are often a fast, safe way to make your smoothies. After all, you don't have to worry if the fruit or vegetables go bad after a month. However, the freezing treatment often means that not all nutrients are the same. Your decision might not make a great deal of difference, but it's important to know what you're getting yourself into.

Fresh fruits and vegetables you would buy at the market are typically picked when they are unripe, and they ripen as they are transported to their destinations. Fruit and vegetables gain their vitamin and mineral value during the trek, which can last as long as a year when stored properly. When you finally bring them home, they usually stay ripe for up to a week.

Frozen fruits and vegetables are harvested when they have reached the peak of ripeness. They are then frozen and soaked in a sugar or ascorbic acid blend that will prevent them from going bad. The most dramatic change in nutrient value occurs in vegetables. To ensure freshness, they are blanched for a few minutes, which can cause them to lose a significant amount of nutrients. Frozen fruits don't go through this treatment and, therefore, retain most of the vitamins and minerals they originally contained. Every company has a different method for freezing fruits, so you could be getting more or fewer nutrients with every serving. Check the label every time you purchase frozen fruit.

So, if you're looking to find a quick alternative to fresh ingredients in your smoothie, consider buying frozen fruit. You can store them for longer without worrying that they'll spoil. However, opt for fresh vegetables. You'll likely get a much richer flavor and you'll ingest more nutrients.

## Step 2: Add Liquid

The liquid you purchase for your smoothies is highly dependent on taste. For example, if you like sweeter smoothies opt for juices, and if you don't want to add calories to your smoothie, substitute the liquid with water. There are also alternatives to these, including coconut water, which gives it an extra punch. As an extra incentive, you can use the bits of coconut you'll find floating in your water for extra flavor!

To make a smoothie creamy, the next step is to add dairy or dairy substitute. Consider adding milk, almond milk, coconut milk, yogurt, or buttermilk to give it extra flavor. Of course, if you're lactose intolerant or simply like the taste of other kinds of milk, you can forego the dairy altogether. Instead, increase the amount of fruit and water or juice to get a similar effect.

## Step 3: Add-Ins

Sometimes the best part of the smoothie isn't the fruit, but what you add to it to give you a thicker, creamier smoothie. These add-ins can also give more nutrition to your meal. For example, adding protein powder will increase your smoothie's thickness and give you a boost of energy until your next meal. Adding white beans or chickpeas, though not typically considered the go-to ingredients for a smoothie, will give your smoothie bulk and give it a salty element.

Consider adding in nut butters as well. You can create smoothies that look and taste like chocolate peanut butter smoothies based on the protein powder and peanut butter you add in. Of course, it takes time to find the perfect matches for your add-ins, so play around with the recipes to get exactly what you want.

## Step 4: Add Ice

One of the best parts of a smoothie is its refreshing coolness, and sometimes the only way to achieve this is by adding ice. In fact, if you pride yourself on using only fresh ingredients, you'll want to invest in an ice tray as well. A colder smoothie can also make you slow down when you eat it, allowing your body to fill up during the meal.

Ice also increases the thickness of your smoothie. If you're looking for a really thick smoothie, consider adding 1 cup or more of crushed ice. If you're using frozen fruit, you can negate the ice as your smoothie will thicken on its own. It's recommended to have a thick smoothie to force you to slow down and enjoy your meal, but it's not necessary. If you want a thinner smoothie, reduce the amount of ice.

# Chapter 3: Fruit and Vegetable Smoothies

Fruits and vegetables are key to a healthy diet, so why wouldn't blending them together be a good idea? If you're struggling to get fruits and vegetables in your diet, consider taking this route. Many people find it difficult to stomach certain types of vegetables, so combining them with your favorite fruits will help you maintain a healthy diet and weight. You'll have all the nutrients you need in a delicious blend. Most of these recipes are under 400 calories!

## Fruit Smoothies

What's better than a refreshing fruit smoothie after a long day of work, or better yet, a snack to wake up to? There's a reason the frozen fruit market has exploded: people are absolutely nuts about fruit smoothies! Test out these delicious recipes and make them your recipe schedule.

*Banana, Berry, and Orange Juice Smoothie*

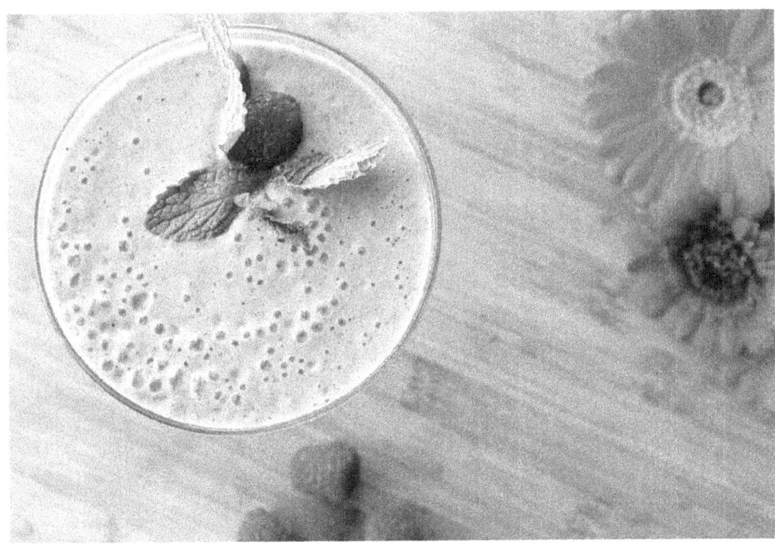

If you're looking for a fun combination of a variety of fruits, look no further. Your smoothie will be a gentle blend of three or more berries combined with banana and orange juice. The juice and natural honey make the smoothie sweet without delving too deeply into pure sugar.

Prep Time: 5 min
Total Time: 5 min
Yield: 2 servings

*Ingredients:*

- 1 frozen or fresh banana
- 2 cups frozen raspberries, cherries, and strawberries
- ½ cup orange juice
- 1 cup milk
- ½ cup vanilla yogurt
- 2 or 3 Tbsp honey
- 2 or 3 ice cubes

*Directions:*

1. First place frozen and fresh fruits and berries in a blender then add orange juice, milk, vanilla yogurt, and honey. Add as many ice cubes as necessary to make the smoothie thicker.
2. Place in the refrigerator until ready to serve.
3. Note: For non-dairy substitutes, substitute almond milk or rice milk for the milk and yogurt.

*Nutrition: 366 calories, 4 g saturated fat, 7 g total fat, 75 g carbohydrates, 88 mg sodium, 6 g fiber, 8 g protein, 58 g sugar*

***Frothy Banana Smoothie***

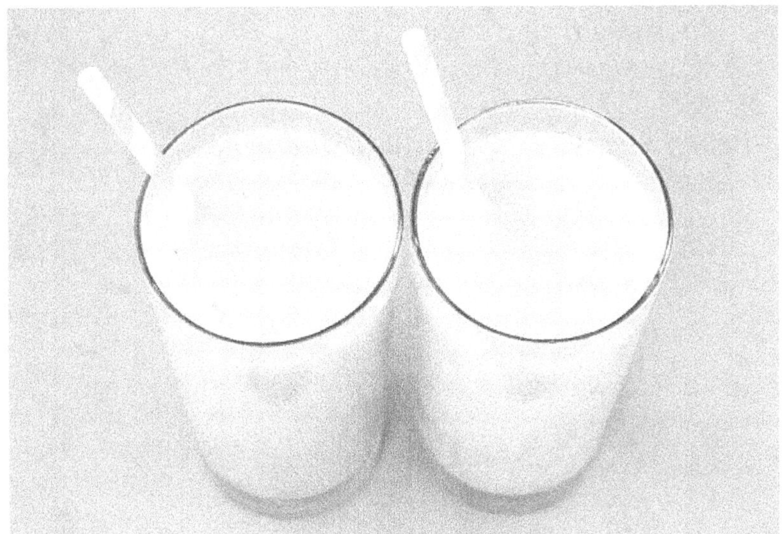

Though the bananas are the star of the show, the addition of strawberries and peaches in this beautiful smoothie gives it that signature Rachel Ray touch. Any berry substitute for strawberry is acceptable, so experiment and find your niche. At only 300 calories per serving, it'll keep you coming back for more.

Prep Time: 8 min
Total Time: 8 min
Yield: 2 servings

*Ingredients:*

- 1 large fresh or frozen banana
- 1 cup sliced peaches, fresh or frozen (frozen peaches should defrost slightly in the microwave before putting in the blender)
- 1 cup fresh or frozen strawberries (frozen strawberries should defrost slightly in the microwave before putting in the blender)
- 1 cup milk
- 1 cup strawberry banana custard yogurt, low fat
- 2 or 3 ice cubes

*Directions:*

1. Defrost all fruit in the microwave until only slightly frozen and break up into smaller pieces with a spoon.
2. Blend on high until smooth and add ice cubes to thicken.
3. Place in the refrigerator until ready to serve.

4. Note: For non-dairy substitutes, consider adding peach juice or almond milk in place of milk and yogurt.

*Nutrition:* 300 calories, 3 g saturated fat, 5 g total fat, 60 g carbohydrates, 127 mg sodium, 3.5 g fiber, 9 g protein, 44 g sugar

### Layered Mango-Peach Strawberry-Banana Smoothie

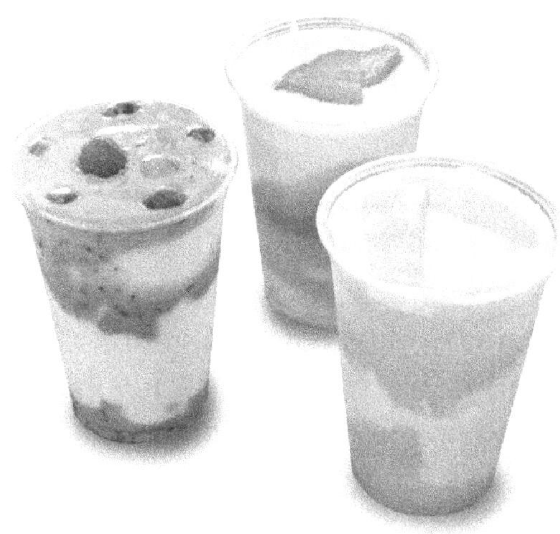

If you're looking for a little more pizazz in your smoothies, consider separating two smoothies to create a single delicious bite. The layered mango peach smoothie combines the two flavors with mango or peach nectar blended with the smooth creaminess of Greek yogurt. Top it off with fresh lime juice and honey.

Prep Time: 30 minutes
Total Time: 1 hr
Yield: 2 servings

*Ingredients Mango-Peach:*

- 1 very ripe peach, peeled, pitted, and sliced
- 1 very ripe mango, peeled, pitted, and sliced
- ½ cup vanilla Greek yogurt
- ½ cup peach or mango nectar
- 1 Tbsp lime juice
- 1 Tbsp honey
- 2 or 3 ice cubes
- Diced mango and peach for garnish

<u>*Ingredients Strawberry Banana:*</u>

- 1 ripe banana, fresh or frozen
- 1 pint strawberries, fresh or frozen, halved
- ½ cup vanilla Greek yogurt
- 1 Tbsp lemon juice
- 1 Tbsp sugar
- 2 or 3 ice cubes
- Diced strawberries for garnish

<u>*Directions:*</u>

1. For the mango-peach smoothie, add fruits, yogurt, and nectar into the blender and blend until smooth. Add lime juice and honey in intervals to get the right consistency. Add ice cubes to add thickness.
2. For the strawberry-banana smoothie, heat strawberries with sugar for 30 minutes and place them in the refrigerator. Add strawberries and banana to a blender, placing yogurt and lemon juice. Add ice cubes to add thickness. Refrigerate when blending is done.
3. Fill glasses half full of each concoction and top with diced fruit.

<u>*Nutrition:*</u> *400 calories, 2 g saturated fat, 4 g total fat, 86 g carbohydrates, 44 mg sodium, 10 g fiber, 16 g protein, 70 g sugar*


**Mango Banana Smoothie**

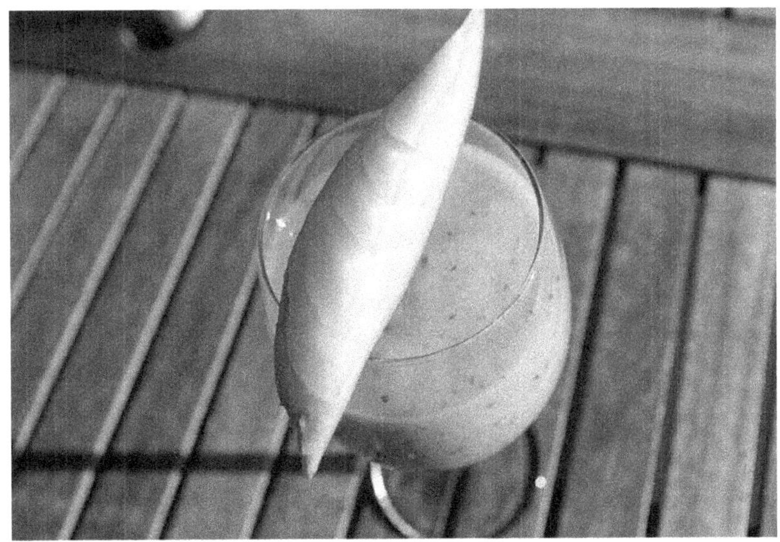

This creamy mango banana smoothie is perfect for those looking for a dairy-free, gluten-free, and vegetarian meal. This smoothie is also great with a wide variety of toppers like chia seeds, pistachios, or fresh blueberries. It's ideal for anyone looking for a quick breakfast, and at only 280 calories, you'll keep coming back for more!

Prep Time: 5 min
Total Time: 5 min
Yield: 2 servings

*Ingredients:*

- 1 banana, fresh or frozen
- 1 cup chopped mango, fresh or frozen
- ¾ cup almond milk
- 2 or 3 ice cubes

*Directions:*

1. First, place the fruit in the blender then add liquids and blend until smooth. Add ice cubes to increase thickness.
2. Place in the refrigerator until ready to serve.

*Nutrition: 280 calories, 16 g saturated fat, 18.5 g total fat, 35 g carbohydrates, 13 mg sodium, 5 g fiber, 3 g protein, 25 g sugar*


**Tropical Smoothie**

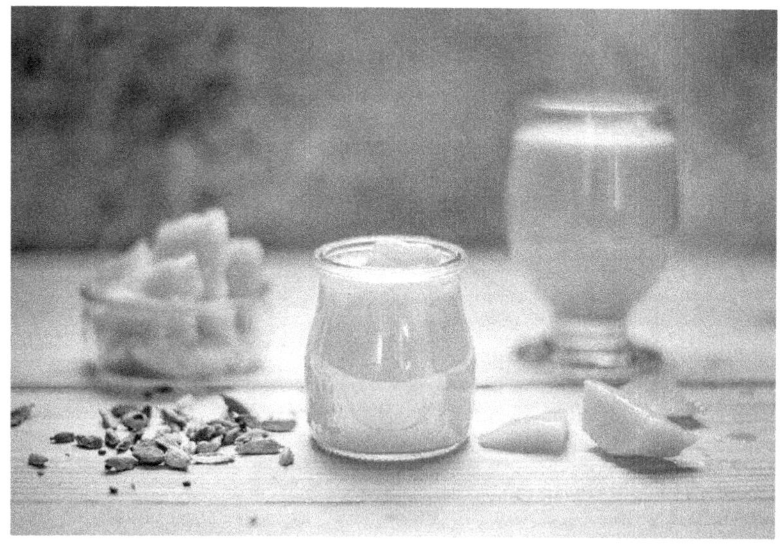

Even if it's nowhere near summer, you'll feel like you're on the beach with this tropical smoothie. Consider eating this smoothie for breakfast and stir in your own granola or chia seeds. This smoothie is highly customizable, so use your favorite fresh or frozen tropical fruit and experiment! This smoothie is only 275 calories, and at only 5 minutes to make, it'll take its place in your morning routine.

Prep Time: 5 min
Total Time: 5 min
Yield: 2 servings

*Ingredients:*

- 1 cup frozen or fresh mango
- 1 cup frozen or fresh pineapple
- 1 kiwi
- ½ banana
- ½ cup coconut milk
- ¼ cup orange juice
- 2 or 3 ice cubes

*Directions:*

1. Add the fruits and orange juice to the blender. Add ice cubes to thicken.
2. Switch up the citrus fruit juice to give a variety of flavors.
3. Place in the refrigerator until ready to serve.

*Nutrition: 275 calories, 13 g fat, 15 g saturated fat, 38 g carbohydrates, 11 mg sodium, 6 g fiber, 3 g protein, 29 g sugar*


# Vegetable Smoothies


Alright, so not everyone is going to love vegetable smoothies, especially if you just throw random vegetables in the blender. Luckily, these vegetable smoothies are the best of the best. You'll be dying to have them for every breakfast. Customize your vegetable smoothies by adding fruits or considering juices.

### *Carrot Smoothie*

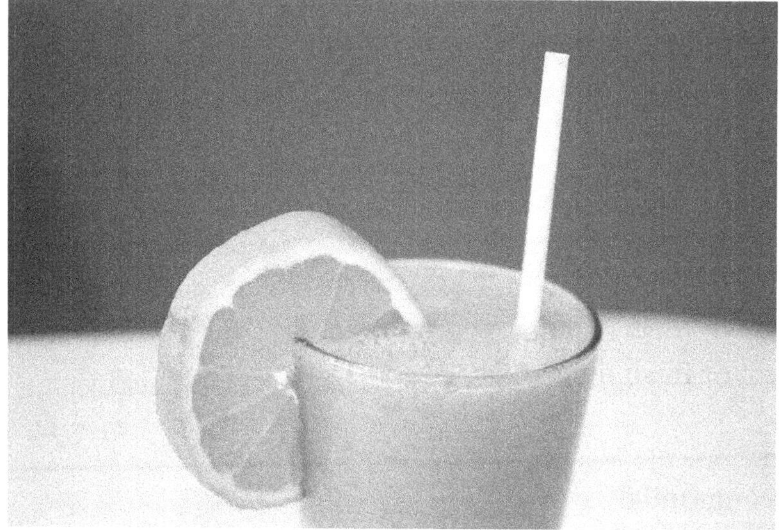

If you're unsure about eating vegetable smoothies, there's no better place to start than with this carrot smoothie. The rich taste of carrot is accentuated with fresh fruits, giving it a beautifully fruity flavor. Carrot is naturally low in calories but loaded with fiber, vitamin C, K, and potassium, and it can improve eye health. At only 185 calories per serving, it's a perfect way to start your day.

Prep Time: 5 min
Total Time: 5 min
Yield: 2 servings

*Ingredients:*

- 1 cup carrots, chopped
- 1 banana, frozen or fresh
- 1 large apple, chopped
- ½ cup pineapple or mango, frozen or fresh
- ½ cup orange juice
- ¼ tsp cinnamon
- 5 ice cubes

*Directions:*

1. Peel carrots and cut them into slices. Chop apples with skins still on and dice fruits.
2. Add to a blender, solids first, then liquids.
3. Place in the refrigerator until ready to serve.

*Nutrition:* 185 calories, 0.5 g saturated fat, 0.7 g total fat, 47 g carbohydrates, 15 mg sodium, 7 g fiber, 2 g protein, 31 g sugar

### Beet Smoothie

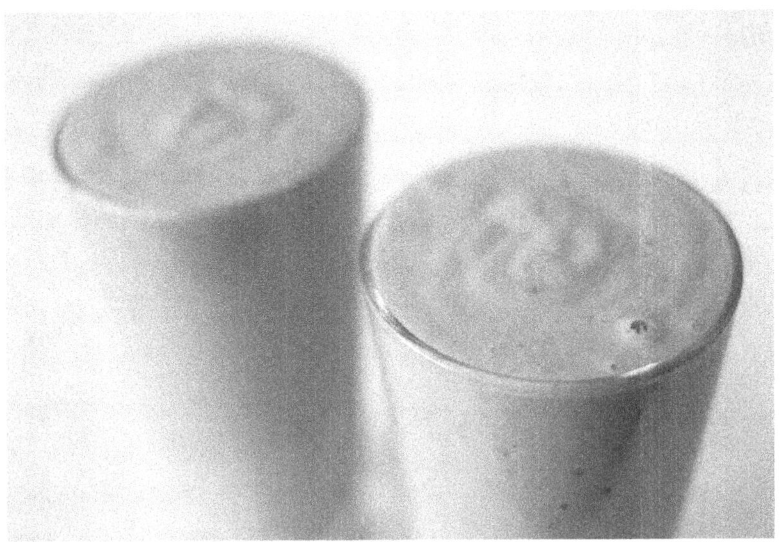

Beets are excellent for you, but they probably don't spend much time in your refrigerator. Luckily, this beet smoothie can give you all the benefits of beets with additional fruity flavors! You can use raw or cooked beets, but be sure you wear gloves because beets will stain your hands.

Prep Time: 5 min
Total Time: 5 min
Yield: 2 servings

*Ingredients:*

- 1 small beet, raw or cooked, room temperature
- 1 banana
- 1 large green apple
- 1 cup frozen mango or pineapple chunks
- ½ cup almond milk or water
- 5 ice cubes

*Directions:*

1. Peel beet and chop. If cooking, let cool to room temperature before placing pieces in the blender. Chop fruit, leaving the skin on the apple.

2. Place all solids into the blender and blend until smooth. Add ice cubes until the smoothie reaches the right consistency.
3. Place in the refrigerator until ready to serve.

*Nutrition:* 150 calories, 0.5 g total fat, 36 g carbohydrate, 20 mg sodium, 5.5 g fiber, 2 g protein, 23 g sugar

## Broccoli Smoothie

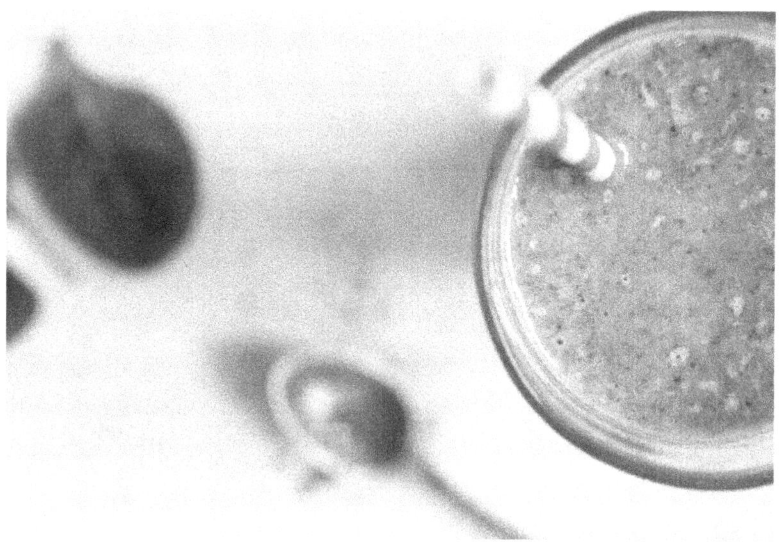

Surprisingly, you can throw broccoli into a blender and make it taste like a fruit smoothie if you add the right ingredients. The combination of banana, apple, pineapple, and yogurt gives this creamy broccoli concoction an amazing flavor while incorporating probiotics, which are helpful for digestion. Consider throwing in some spices to make this smoothie your own!

Prep Time: 5 min
Total Time: 5 min
Yield: 2 servings

*Ingredients:*

- 1 cup broccoli florets, chopped
- 1 banana, fresh or frozen
- 1 large green apple, chopped
- 1 cup pineapple, fresh or frozen, chopped
- ½ cup water
- ½ cup vanilla Greek yogurt

<u>*Directions:*</u>

1. Add solids to the blender, then add water and vanilla Greek yogurt, blending until smooth.
2. Place in the refrigerator until ready to serve.

<u>*Nutrition:*</u> *270 calories, 0.8 g saturated fat, 1.7 g total fat, 61 g carbohydrate, 37 mg sodium, 7 g fiber, 8 g protein, 47 g sugar*


## Pumpkin Smoothie

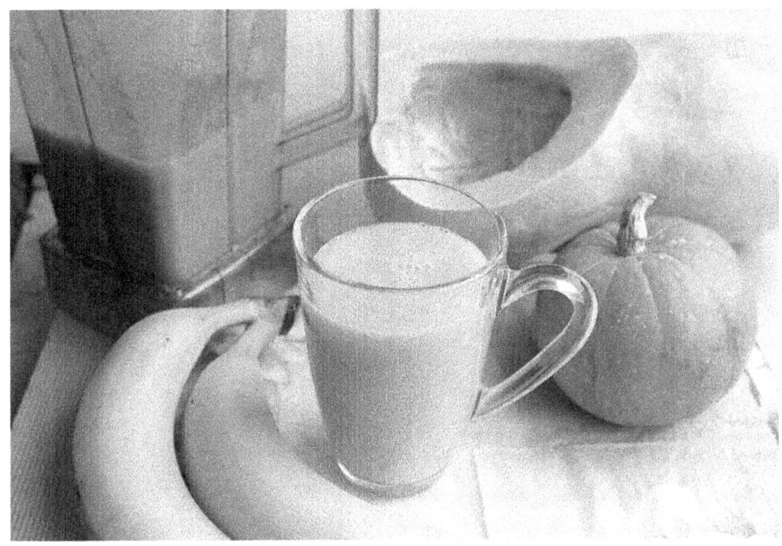

Even if it's not Halloween season, jump into a delicious pumpkin smoothie. Unlike most pumpkin desserts over the holidays, this pumpkin smoothie isn't loaded with sugar, and it has a punch of protein from the yogurt. Of course, you'll need to add a little bit of sweetness to the smoothie, so indulge in a little bit of maple syrup.

Prep Time: 5 min

Total Time: 5 min

Yield: 2 servings

<u>*Ingredients:*</u>

- ½ cup pumpkin puree
- 1 ½ cup fresh apple chunks, chopped with skin on
- 1 banana
- 1 tsp pumpkin spice

- ½ cup vanilla Greek yogurt
- 1 tsp vanilla extract
- 1 ½ Tbsp maple syrup
- 5 ice cubes
- Maple granola

*Directions:*

1. Add all solids into the blender, gently stirring. Break banana into pieces in the blender. Add liquids and blend until smooth, occasionally scraping the sides of the blender
2. Add water as necessary to reduce thickness.
3. Place in the refrigerator until ready to serve.

*Nutrition: 275 calories, 1 g saturated fat, 2 g total fat, 62 g carbohydrates, 24 mg sodium, 9 g fiber, 7 g protein, 44 g sugar*

# Chapter 4: Berry Smoothies

A little bit of berry smoothie goes a long way. There's a reason that people love to eat berry smoothies: they have some of the best-tasting recipes. Frozen berries are easy to acquire, and they are easy to fit into a small container. And, with no added preservatives, you don't have to feel like you don't know what's going into your stomach.

Berries contain a lot of natural sugars, so it's easy to go overboard with your favorite recipes, but know what to say yes to. For example, instead of choosing juices, stick to water, almond milk, coconut milk, or yogurt. Remember to never overindulge in berry smoothies. You may start to feel sick consuming so much natural sugar.

This chapter contains some of the most classic berry smoothies you could find, but you'll also likely find recipes for berries you would never consider. Each has its own wide variety of health benefits, so load up on some of your favorite smoothies!

***Mixed Berry Smoothie***

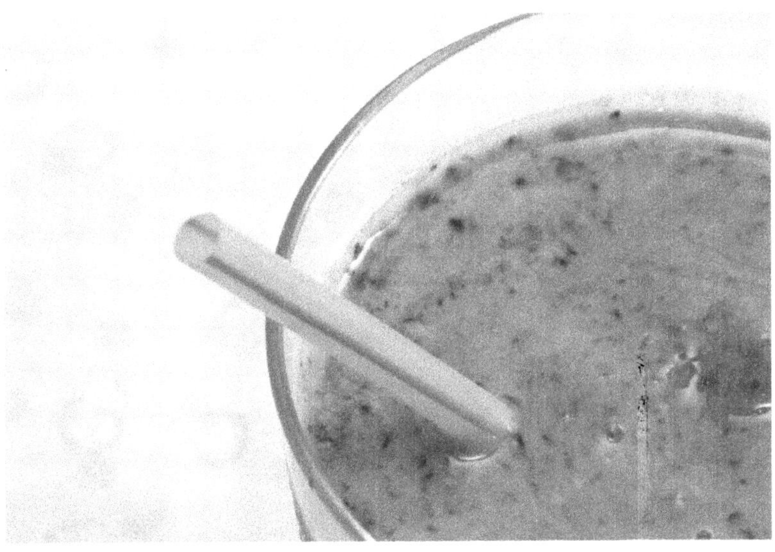

The mixed berry smoothie is a favorite because it is so delicious. Berries are loaded with antioxidants, vitamins, and fiber, which are vital ingredients that are not as readily available in common meals. As a bonus, the protein from the Greek yogurt will keep you feeling full until lunchtime!

Prep Time: 5 min
Total Time: 5 min

Yield: 2 servings

*Ingredients:*

- 1 banana, cut in chunks
- 1 ½ cup mixed berries, frozen
- 1 ½ cup apple juice (replace with almond milk or coconut milk to lower total calorie number)
- ¾ cup vanilla Greek yogurt
- 2 or 3 ice cubes
- 1 Tbsp honey

*Directions:*

1. Add all solid ingredients to the blender followed by liquids. Add more liquid to vary the smoothie thickness. Add ice cubes to increase thickness.
2. Stir in honey to your liking and place mixed berries as a garnish on top.
3. Place in the refrigerator until ready to serve.

*Nutrition: 220 calories, 0.5 g saturated fat, 1 g total fat, 52 g carbohydrates, 60 mg sodium, 4 g fiber, 6 g protein, 41 g sugar*


**Strawberry Smoothie**

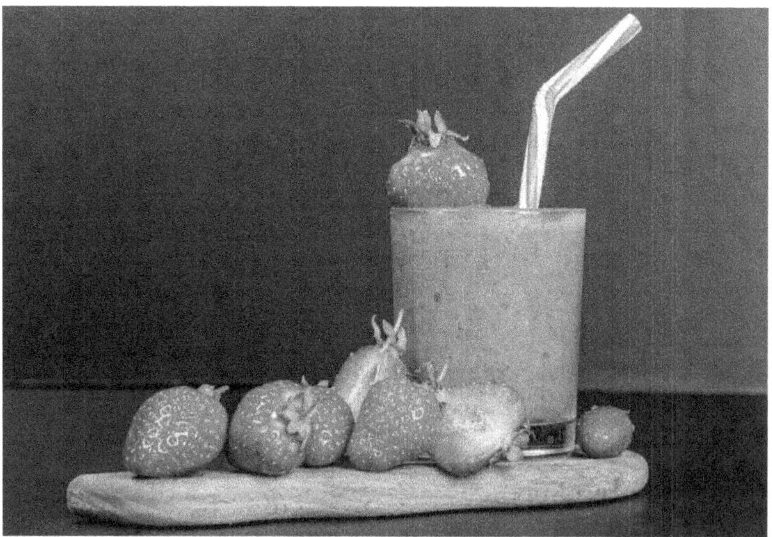

Nothing is better than a classic strawberry smoothie. Some recipes can feel overly complicated, but sometimes all you need is a classic strawberry smoothie. This recipe takes only three ingredients and is done in a matter of minutes. Plus, if you're feeling adventurous, you can always add a variety of jams and jellies to switch up the flavors. With only 170 calories, this smoothie will be a go-to from now on.

Prep Time: 5 min
Total Time: 5 min
Yield: 2 servings

*Ingredients:*

- 1 ½ cup strawberries, fresh or frozen
- ¾ cup milk (you can use almond milk or coconut milk as a replacement)
- ¼ cup strawberry jam
- 2 or 3 ice cubes

*Direction:*

1. Place all solid foods into the blender, then add liquids. Blend until smooth. Add ice cubes to increase thickness.
2. Place in the refrigerator until ready to serve.

*Nutrition: 170 calories, 3 g saturated fat, 3 g total fat, 32 g carbohydrates, 50 mg sodium, 2 g fiber, 32 g protein, 2 g sugar*


**Raspberry Smoothie**

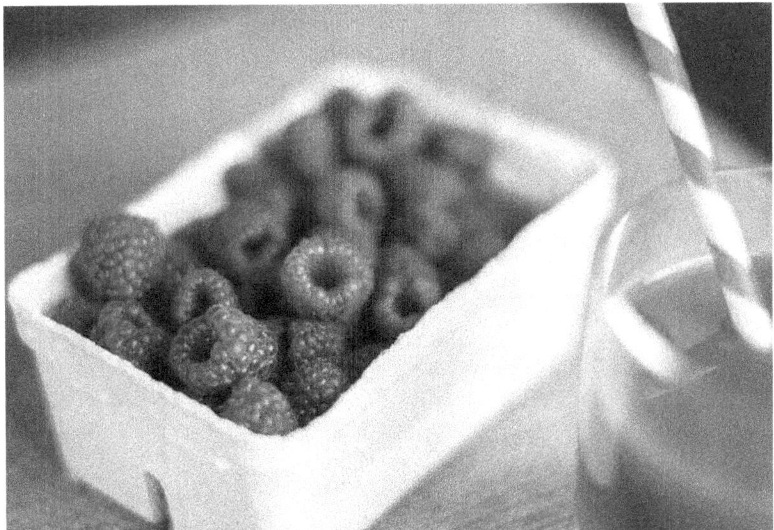

Raspberries are rich in vitamin C and delicious. Just like the other recipes, you can replace raspberries with other berries, but why would you want to? This smoothie is beautiful, and an added mint leaf garnish gives it an extra kick. At only 225 calories, it's a favorite in this book.

Prep Time: 5 min
Total Time: 5 min
Yield: 2 servings

*Ingredients:*

- 1 ½ cup raspberries, fresh or frozen
- 1 banana, chopped
- 1 ½ cup apple juice (consider replacing with almond milk or water for a lower calorie count)
- ¾ cup vanilla Greek yogurt
- 2 or 3 ice cubes
- 1 Tbsp honey

*Directions:*

1. Add solid foods first, then add liquids and blend until smooth. Add ice cubes to increase thickness.
2. Place in the refrigerator until ready to serve.

*Nutrition: 225 calories, 1 g saturated fat, 1 g total fat, 34 g carbohydrates, 34 mg sodium, 7 g fiber, 8 g protein, 27 g sugar*


**Blackberry Smoothie**

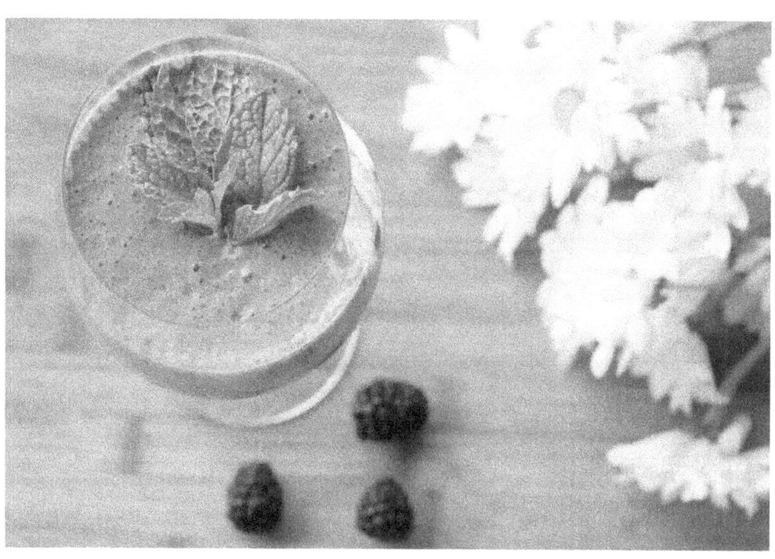

Blackberries are some of the best berries to come out of the bush. They offer a wide variety of nutrients including vitamins A, C, E, potassium, and calcium, among others. Although it's impossible to say that one berry can act as a superfood that can cure a variety of ills, blackberry studies have found connections between increased blackberry consumption and a reduced risk of heart disease and cancer. Blackberries have also been found to improve brainpower. So, consider adding this superfood smoothie to your weekly routine.

Prep Time: 5 min
Total Time: 5 min
Yield: 2 servings

*Ingredients:*

- 1 ½ cup blackberries, fresh or frozen
- 1 cup pineapple chunks, fresh or frozen
- 1 cup vanilla, non-fat Greek yogurt
- 2 cups milk (replace with almond milk or coconut milk)
- 2 or 3 ice cubes
- 2 Tbsp honey

*Directions:*

1. Add solid food to the blender followed by liquids and blend until smooth. Add ice cubes to increase thickness.
2. Place in the refrigerator until ready to serve.

*Nutrition: 180 calories, 1 g saturated fat, 5 g total fat, 34 g carbohydrates, 410 mg sodium, 10 g fiber, 4 g protein, 24 g sugar*

***Blueberry Smoothie***

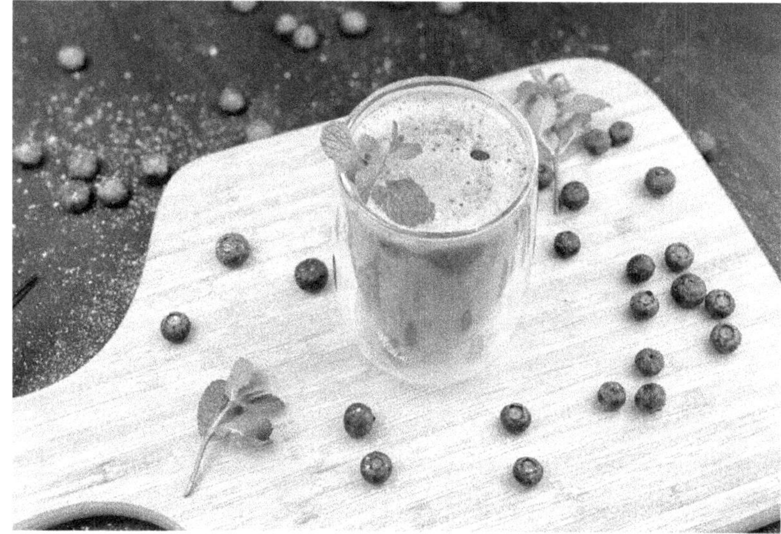

Blueberries can be added to nearly every food and are widely popular. Blueberries only have a few calories per serving, but they are rich in fiber, manganese, vitamins C and K, and a wide variety of other nutrients (Leech, 2018). Blueberries are also rich in antioxidants, which aid in replacing cells. Blueberries can also reduce bad cholesterol in your body, which means they are beneficial for those with heart problems. Whatever your reason for wanting a blueberry smoothie, you'll not find a better recipe than this.

Prep Time: 5 min
Total Time: 5 min
Yield: 2 servings

*Ingredients:*

- 1 cup blueberries, fresh or frozen
- 8 oz vanilla yogurt
- ¾ cup almond milk
- 2 Tbsp sugar
- ½ tsp vanilla extract
- ½ tsp ground nutmeg
- 2 or 3 ice cubes

*Directions:*

1. Add solid foods first then add liquids. Smoothie will become brothy, so scrape the edges of the blender frequently. Add ice cubes to increase thickness.
2. Place in the refrigerator until ready to serve.

*Nutrition:* 210 calories, 2.4 g saturated fat, 4 g total fat, 35 g carbohydrates, 118 g sodium, 2 g fiber, 10 g protein, 32 g sugar

## Cranberry Smoothie

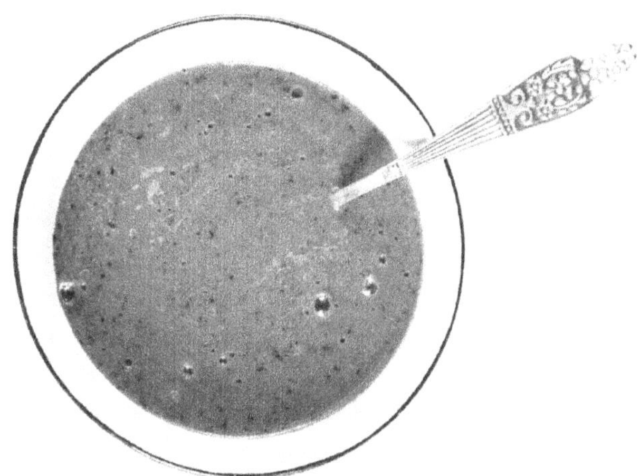

You can truly make a smoothie out of anything. Cranberries are excellent for your health because they are high in fiber and low in fat. They contain manganese, vitamin C, E, and K, and copper. Cranberry juice is commonly used for urinary tract infections, but cranberries also improve eyesight, lower blood pressure, and improve cardiovascular health, among other benefits (Pathak, 2020). This healing smoothie should remain in your recipe book to make you feel better.

Prep Time: 5 min
Total Time: 5 min
Yield: 2 servings

*Ingredients:*

- 8 oz whole cranberries, fresh or frozen
- 1 banana, fresh or frozen
- 2 oranges, peeled
- 2 Tbsp maple syrup
- ½ cup water
- 2 or 3 ice cubes

*Directions:*

1. Place solid foods into the blender first, then add liquids, and blend until smooth. Add ice cubes to increase thickness.
2. Adjust the amount of maple syrup to your liking for a more tart or sweet result.

*Nutrients:* 215 calories, 0.1 g saturated fat, 0.5 total fat, 55 g carbohydrate, 2 mg sodium, 8 g fiber, 3 g protein, 40 g sugar


### Boysenberry-Banana Smoothie

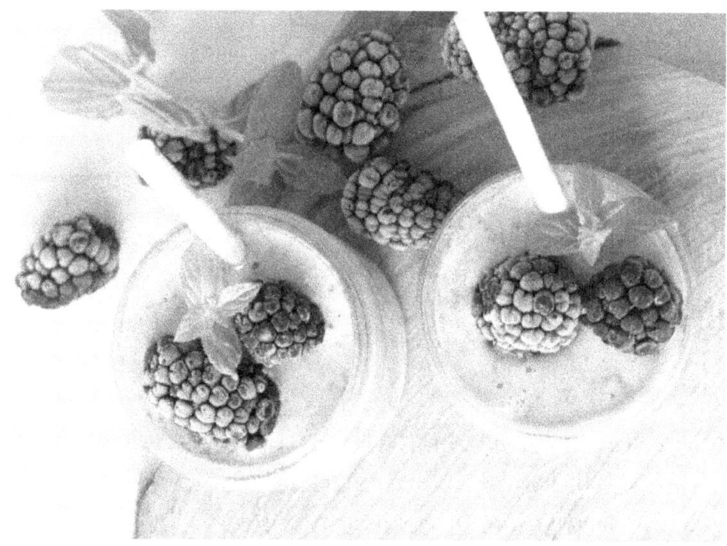

Many people probably haven't heard of boysenberries, but it's time you added them to your shopping list. Boysenberries are low in calories, and they are commonly used in salads because they are low in fat, making them perfect for weight loss. Boysenberries are also helpful in creating beautiful, fresh skin and aid in brain health. At only 150 calories, you'll keep reaching for this in the future.

Prep Time: 5 min
Total Time: 5 min
Yield: 2 servings

*Ingredients:*

- ¾ cup boysenberries, fresh or frozen
- ½ banana, sliced
- ½ cup boysenberry yogurt
- ½ cup cherry or grape juice
- 2 or 3 ice cubes

*Directions:*

1. Add solid foods first, then add liquids, and blend until smooth. Add ice cubes to increase thickness.
2. Place in the refrigerator until ready to serve.

*Nutrition:* *150 calories, 0.5 g saturated fat, 1 g total fat, 32.5 g carbohydrate, 40 mg sodium, 3 g fiber, 4 g protein, 25 g sugar*

## Huckleberry Smoothie

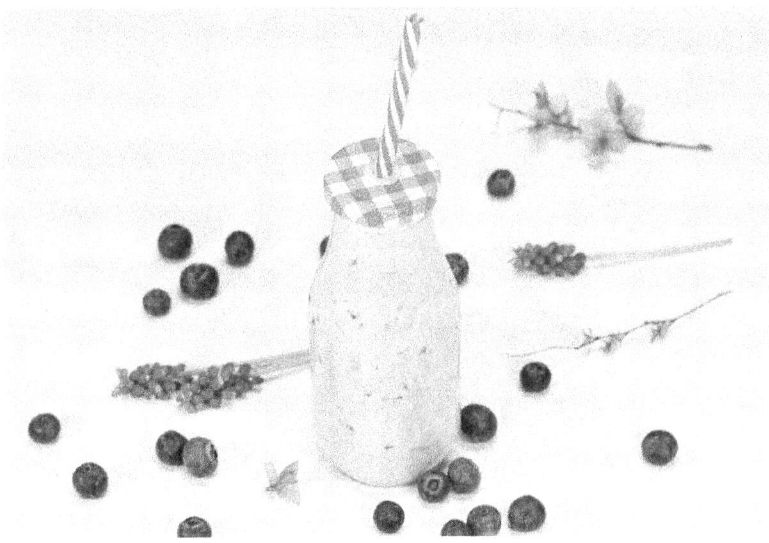

Huckleberries are a delicacy of the Rocky Mountains, and you'll find that people out west have a great love for them, and rightly so. Huckleberries are incredibly delicious and healthy. Huckleberries are loaded with antioxidants, which aid in heart health and can lower blood pressure. They are also rich in iron, giving your blood an extra boost. You may also notice that huckleberries are commonly used in natural remedies for infections because they contain a lot of vitamin C. So if you've never tried huckleberries in your smoothies, it's time to start.

Prep Time: 5 min
Total Time: 5 min
Yield: 2 servings

*Ingredients:*

- 1 banana, sliced
- 1 ½ cup huckleberries, fresh or frozen

- 2 cups almond milk
- 1 Tbsp rice protein
- ½ tsp ground cinnamon
- 2 or 3 ice cubes

*Directions:*

1. Add solid foods first, then add liquids, and blend until smooth. Gradually add cinnamon to your liking. Add ice cubes to increase thickness.
2. Place in the refrigerator until ready to serve.

*Nutrition:* 215 calories, 0.1 g saturated fat, 4 g total fat, 40 g carbohydrate, 145 mg sodium, 5 g fiber, 9 g protein, 24 g sugar


## Elderberry Smoothie

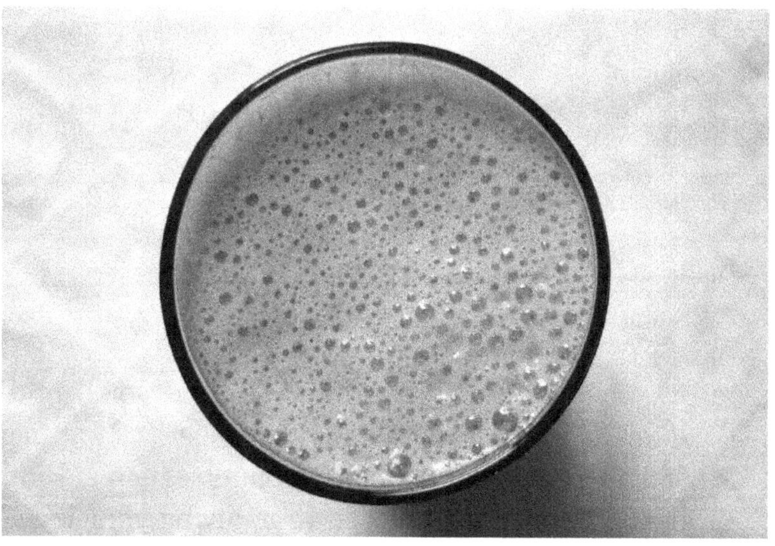

Elderberries are not just a *Monty Python and the Holy Grail* reference; they actually have quite a following. Elderberries have been used throughout history to treat wounds, heal burns, and improve skin health. Elderberries are high in vitamin C, fiber, and antioxidants. These benefits can aid in healing flu symptoms, and they, like those berries listed above, are useful in maintaining heart health. If you're looking for something a little exotic, head over to your grocery store and use elderberries.

Prep Time: 5 min
Total Time: 5 min
Yield: 2 servings

_Ingredients:_

- ½ cup elderberry juice
- 1 large grapefruit
- ½ cup mangos, fresh or frozen
- ½ cup raspberries, fresh or frozen
- 1 cup blueberries, fresh or frozen
- ¼ cup water
- 2 or 3 ice cubes

_Directions:_

1. Add solid foods into the blender first, squeezing only the grapefruit juice into the blender. Next, add liquids, blending until smooth. Add ice cubes to increase thickness.
2. Place in the refrigerator until ready to serve.

_Nutrition: 200 calories, 0 g saturated fat, 0.7 g total fat, 52 g carbohydrate, 3 mg sodium, 9 g fiber, 3 g protein, 37 g sugar_


**Black Currant Smoothie**

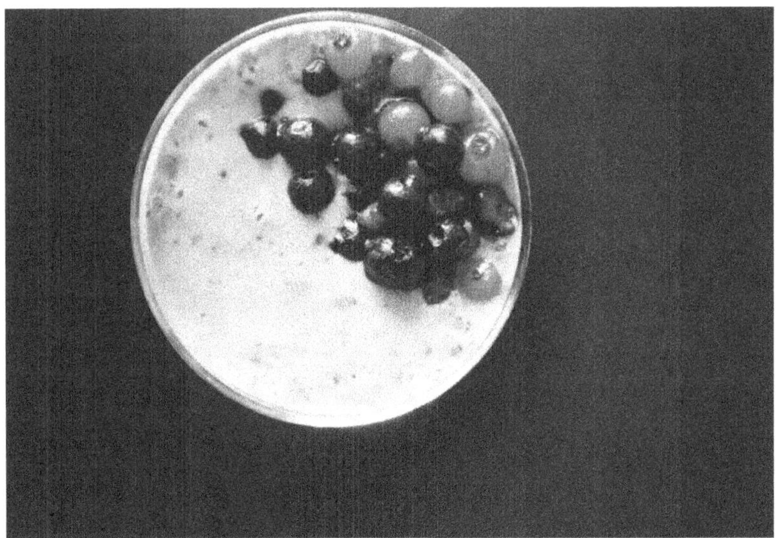

You're not likely to see a lot of black currant recipes if you live in the United States. The berries were originally considered a fungus and weed, but have become a favorite in jams and juices. Black currants are vitamin superstars, containing vitamins A, C, E, and almost all B vitamins. Because of this, black currants are common for immune system help and could have possible anti-cancer properties. So, delve into black currants with this delicious recipe.

Prep Time: 5 min
Total Time: 5 min
Yield: 2 servings

*Ingredients:*

- 1 cup black currants, fresh or frozen
- ½ cup strawberries, fresh or frozen
- ½ cup coconut milk
- 1 cup water
- 1 tsp vanilla extract
- 2 or 3 ice cubes

*Directions:*

1. Add all berries then liquids, and blend until smooth. Add ice cubes to increase thickness.
2. Place in the refrigerator until ready to serve.

*Nutrition: 230 calories, 11.2 g saturated fat, 17.3 g total fat, 17.2 g carbohydrate, 19 mg sodium, 8.5 g fiber, 5.1 g protein, 6 g sugar*


**Mulberry Smoothie**

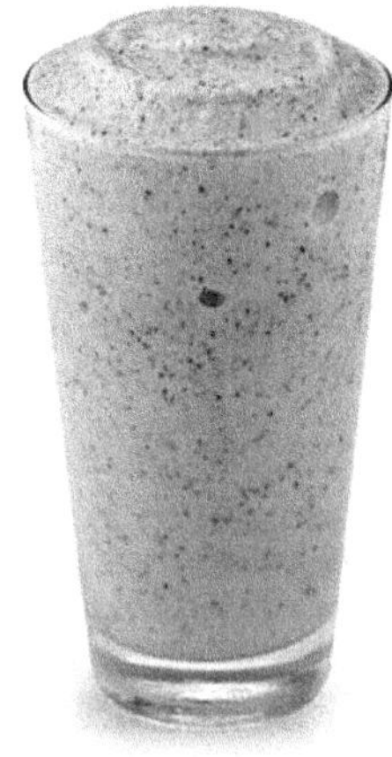

Mulberries aren't just the subject of a classic nursery rhyme; they're also nutritious berries that make perfect breakfast smoothies. Like the other berries listed here, mulberries are chock full of vitamins, including vitamin C, E, and K, and they also contain high levels of potassium and iron. This smoothie is low in fat and high in protein, perfect for getting you through until lunch.

Prep Time: 5 min
Total Time: 5 min
Yield: 2 servings

*Ingredients:*

- 1 cup mulberries, fresh
- 1 banana
- 1 cup vanilla Greek yogurt
- ¼ cup whole oats
- ½ cup almond milk
- 1 Tbsp chia seeds
- 2 or 3 ice cubes

*Directions:*

1. Add solid ingredients to the blender first, then add liquid ingredients and blend until smooth. Add ice cubes to increase thickness.
2. Place in the refrigerator until ready to serve.

*Nutrition: 380 calories, 14 g saturated fat, 19 g total fat, 45 g carbohydrate, 43 mg sodium, 7.5 g fiber, 12.5 g protein, 23.5 g sugar*

# Chapter 5: Combo Smoothies

Combo smoothies combine a wide variety of fruits, vegetables, and berries, giving some of the best-tasting smoothies out there. Combining smoothies with an array of spices and unusual ingredients can also give you more health benefits than sticking strictly to common fruits and vegetables. If you're in the mood to try something outside the box, make these delicious smoothies with less than 300 calories and a total prep time of five minutes!

### *Wheatgrass Apple Smoothie*

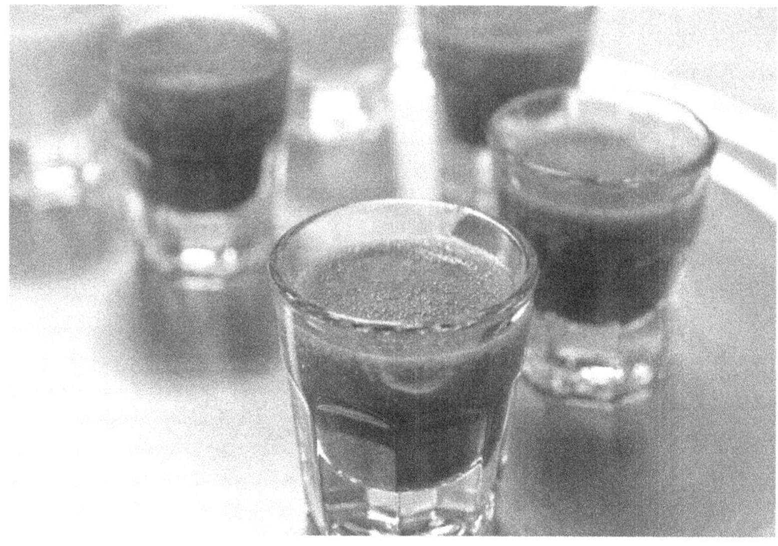

Not for the smoothie newbie, this wheatgrass smoothie has a more earthy taste than most other smoothies. Wheatgrass is often introduced as a superfood due to its abundance of enzymes, vitamins, and minerals, and it is often used as a way to remove toxins from the body. According to Healthline's Emily Cronkleton (2017), wheatgrass has been proven as a way to boost metabolism and reduce cravings. Though this smoothie may be an acquired taste, it's certainly worth putting it on your weekly smoothie schedule.

Prep Time: 5 min
Total Time: 5 min
Yield: 2 servings

*Ingredients:*

- 2 handfuls of fresh baby spinach leaves
- 1 handful of fresh baby kale leaves
- ¼ cup mango chunks, fresh or frozen
- ¼ cup raspberries, fresh or frozen
- 1 ½ tsp wheatgrass powder
- 1 cup apple juice
- ¼ cup pomegranate juice
- 2 or 3 ice cubes

*Directions:*

1. Add all frozen foods together then add liquid ingredients and blend until smooth. Add ice cubes to increase thickness.
2. Place in the refrigerator until ready to serve.

*Nutrition: 300 calories, 0.1 g saturated fat, 1 g total fat, 63 g carbohydrate, 155 mg sodium, 5.3 g fiber, 5.5 g protein, 51 g sugar*


## Acai Power Smoothie Bowl

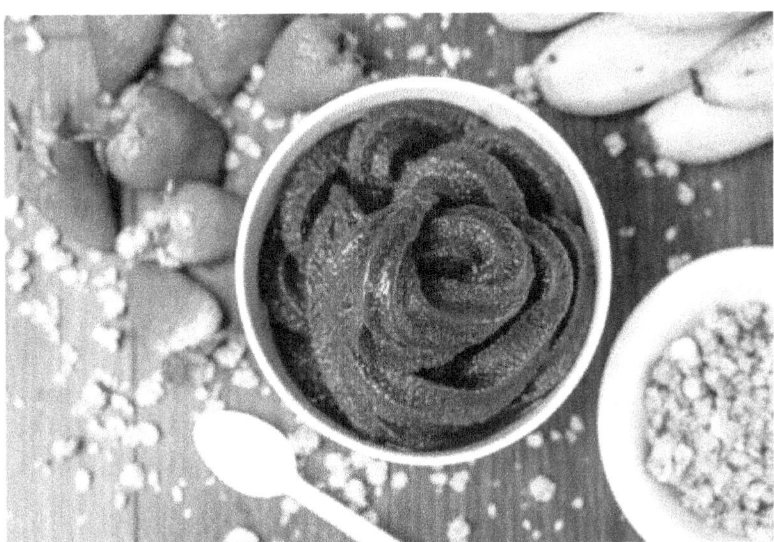

Acai berries have exploded in popularity in the past decade, partially because they're considered a superfruit. Like most berries, acai berries are loaded with antioxidants, which are responsible for maintaining healthy skin and prevent diseases. They are also attributed to aiding brainpower. So, if you want to start your day right, make the most of this acai power smoothie bowl.

Prep Time: 5 min

Total Time: 10 min
Yield: 2 servings

*Ingredients:*

- 2, 4-oz packets unsweetened acai puree
- 2 Medjool dates, pitted
- ½ cup strawberries, fresh or frozen
- ½ cup mangos, fresh or frozen
- ½ cup kale leaves
- 1 banana
- ¾ cup almond milk
- ¼ cup vanilla Greek yogurt
- 1 Tbsp lime juice
- 2 tsp maca powder
- 2 or 3 ice cubes

*Directions:*

1. Crush acai berries with a rolling pin. Pour milk in the blender then add solid foods and blend until smooth, occasionally stopping to scrape sides. Don't over-blend, which will cause the smoothie to thin.
2. Pour smoothie mixture into bowls and refrigerate until ready to serve.
3. Note: Adding toppings such as goji berries or granola are great additions.

*Nutrition: 455 calories, 2.6 g saturated fat, 7 g total fat, 75 g carbohydrate, 155 mg sodium, 9 g fiber, 27 g protein, 42 g sugar*

***Roasted Strawberry and Tahini Smoothie***

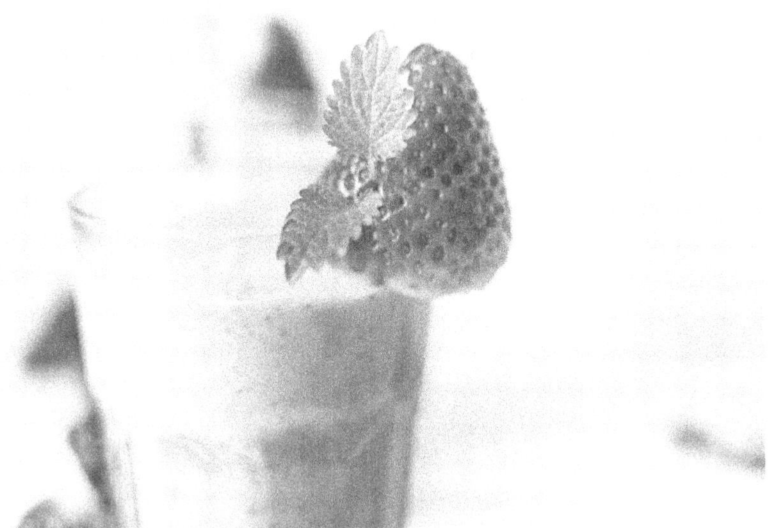

Tahini is ground sesame seeds and is commonly used in hummus, but it's likely you've never heard of some of the best elements of it. Tahini is loaded with thiamine, phosphorus, and manganese, among other vitamins and minerals. It's also a common method for treating bacterial infections, as it has antibacterial properties. This smoothie may seem unusual, but it may just become your favorite go-to smoothie to make you feel great.

Prep Time: 5 min
Total Time: 30 min
Yield: 2 servings

*Ingredients:*

- 2 cups strawberries
- 3 Tbsp sugar
- 1 banana, frozen
- 3 Tbsp tahini
- ½ cup buttermilk
- 2 or 3 ice cubes

*Directions:*

1. Preheat oven to 400°. Combine strawberries and sugar onto baking sheet. Roast strawberries until soft, or 20-25 min and let cool.
2. Transfer ¾ of strawberries in a blender with the rest of the ingredients and blend until smooth.

3.  Smash remaining strawberries into a paste and stir into smoothie.
4.  Place in the refrigerator until ready to serve.

*Nutrition:* *360 calories, 2 g saturated fat, 13.5 g total fat, 59 g carbohydrate, 93 mg sodium, 8.4 g fiber, 8 g protein, 40.5 g sugar*

## CBD Mango Smoothie

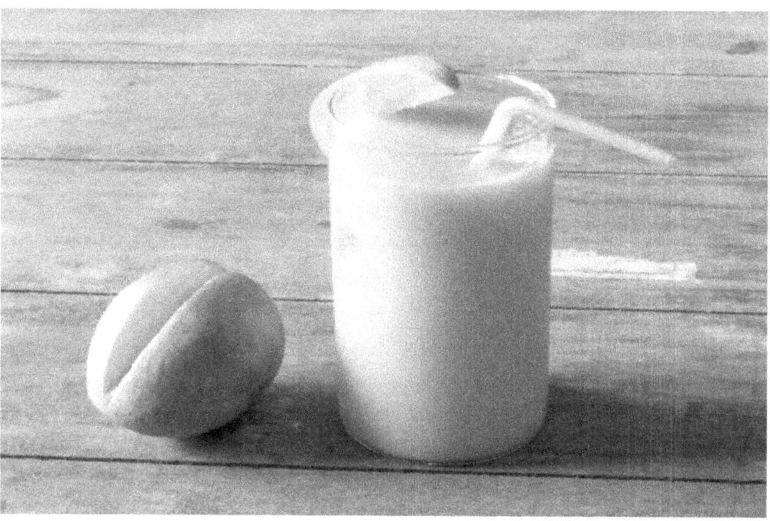

With the legalization of marijuana in many states, people have been on opposite sides of the spectrum when it comes to its consumption. There have been many health benefits associated with marijuana, but it is still highly controversial. Luckily, cannabidiol (CBD) has the same healing properties of marijuana without the hallucinogenic properties. So, people have been running to this pain-relieving wonder.

CBD oil has gone through several studies to determine its complete benefits. In one study, Brazilian men took either a CBD pill or a placebo, and the results concluded that CBD was beneficial in reducing depression and anxiety. It's also been tested as a method to reduce the effects of insomnia. If you've yet to jump on the CBD bandwagon, it's about time you did.

Prep Time: 5 min
Total Time: 5 min
Yield: 2 servings

*Ingredients:*

*   1 mango, peeled and chopped

- 1 banana
- 1-inch piece of ginger, peeled and grated
- ½ tsp CBD oil
- ½ tsp ground turmeric
- ½ cup coconut water
- 2 or 3 ice cubes

*Directions:*

1. Place all solid ingredients in blender then add liquids and blend until smooth. Add ice cubes to increase thickness.
2. Place in the refrigerator until ready to serve.

*Nutrition: 250 calories, 0.3 g saturated fat, 4 g total fat, 56 g carbohydrate, 73 mg sodium, 4.5 g fiber, 2 g protein, 45 g sugar*

## Blueberry Cashew Smoothie

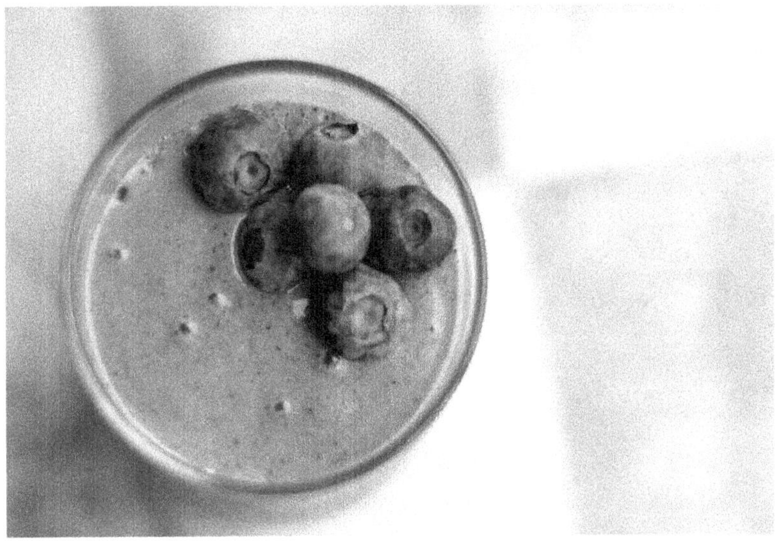

Those looking for an alternative protein source that is also high in a variety of vitamins and minerals will love this blueberry cashew smoothie. It is low in sugar and high in unsaturated fats, keeping you feeling full for longer. Cashews are also linked to weight loss because they are highly fibrous and allow your body to absorb more of the nutrients as they travel through the body. Dive into this delicious blueberry cashew smoothie to promote your future weight loss journey!

Prep Time: 5 min
Total Time: 5 min

Yield: 2 servings

*Ingredients:*

- ½ cup cashews
- ½ cup blueberries, fresh or frozen
- 1 Medjool date, pitted
- 1 cup unsweetened coconut water
- ⅓ cup vanilla Greek yogurt
- ½ Tbsp lime juice
- 2 or 3 ice cubes

*Directions:*

1. Place solid ingredients in blender first followed by wet ingredients and blend until smooth. Add ice cubes to increase thickness.
2. Place in the refrigerator until ready to serve.

*Nutrition: 340 calories, 3.5 g saturated fat, 16.5 g total fat, 45 g carbohydrate, 135 mg sodium, 5.3 g fiber, 8.6 g protein, 28 g sugar*


## Almond Banana Smoothie

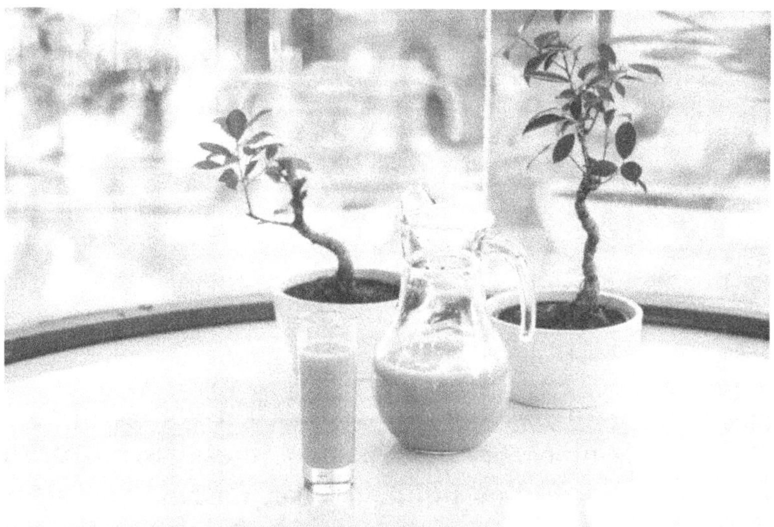

Almonds are available in granola, fancy dishes, and even chocolate. They are massively popular around the world because of their great taste, but they're also packed with tons of nutrients. These small nuts contain a lot of protein, fiber, and healthy fats that help other nutrients to be easily digested. Almonds have been proven to lower blood pressure and aid in the digestion of insulin in people with type 2 diabetes. But, even if you're just in it for the taste, this almond banana smoothie will keep you coming back for more!

Prep Time: 5 min
Total Time: 5 min
Yield: 2 servings

*Ingredients:*

- 1 banana, fresh or frozen
- 1 cup almond milk
- 1 Tbsp almond butter
- 2 or 3 ice cubes

*Directions:*

1. Place banana in blender then incorporate almond milk and butter and blend until smooth. Add ice cubes to increase thickness.
2. Place in the refrigerator until ready to serve.

*Nutrition: 130 calories, 0.6 g saturated fat, 6.5 g total fat, 18 g carbohydrate, 90 mg sodium, 3 g fiber, 3 g protein, 8.7 g sugar*


## Honeydew Cucumber Smoothie

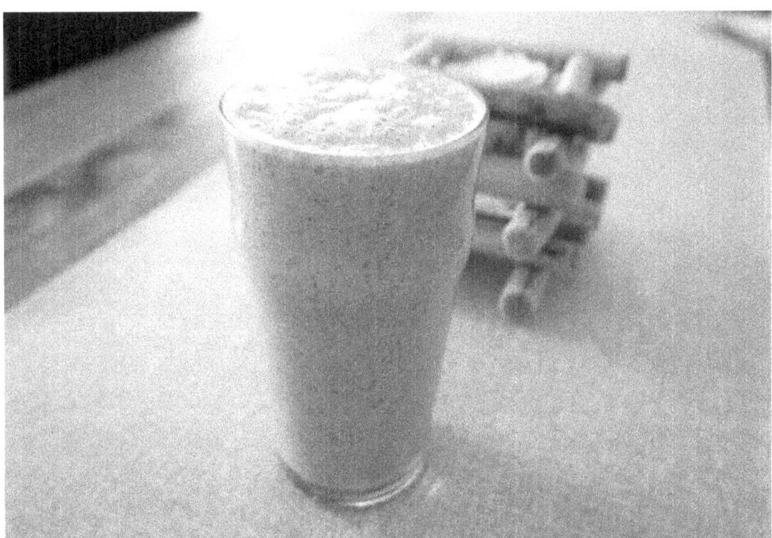

Though melons are notorious for being mostly water, they are packed with nutrients for healthy living, including bone health. Over time, bones become more porous, but vitamins and minerals such as folate, magnesium, and vitamin K are responsible for increasing their density. Honeydew will also give you more glowing skin because it's rich in vitamin C.

Prep Time: 5 min
Total Time: 5 min
Yield: 2 servings

*Ingredients:*

- 2 ⅔ cup honeydew melon, fresh or frozen
- 2 cup coconut water
- 4 tsp lime juice
- 4 oz cucumber, peeled and sliced
- 2 or 3 ice cubes

*Directions:*

1. Add solid ingredients then add liquids and blend until smooth. Add ice cubes to increase thickness.
2. Place in the refrigerator until ready to serve.

*Nutrition: 150 calories, 0.5 g saturated fat, 1 g total fat, 36 g carbohydrate, 300 mg sodium, 5 g fiber, 3.5 g protein, 27 g sugar*


**Carrot, Turmeric, and Ginger Smoothie**

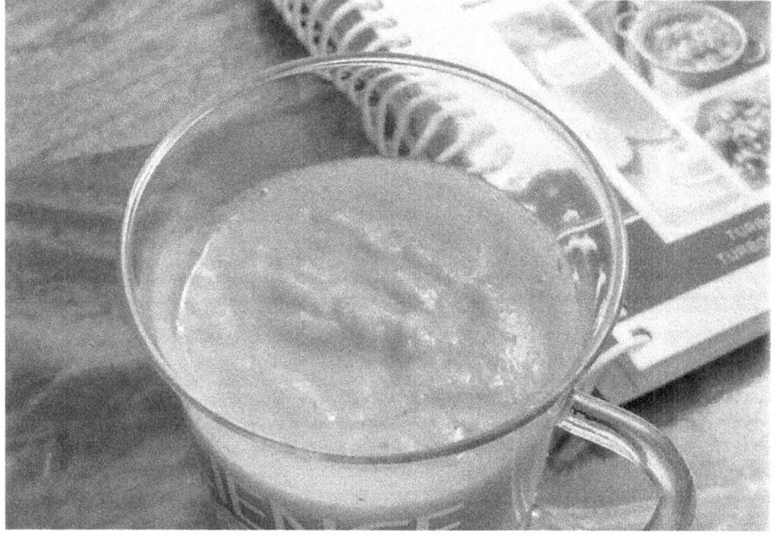

If you've only just heard of the health benefits of ginger and turmeric, you're likely behind the times. Originating in China, both ginger and turmeric have been used as both spices and medicinal additives for thousands of years. Ginger and Turmeric are natural anti-inflammatory agents that can improve pains ranging from menstruation to arthritis. If you're feeling bloated or nauseous, keep these ingredients in your pantry: they're known for calming a bristling stomach.

Prep Time: 5 min
Total Time: 5 min
Yield: 2 servings

*Ingredients:*

- 1 carrot, scrubbed
- 1 orange, peeled
- ½ cup mango, fresh or frozen
- ⅔ cup unsweetened coconut water
- ¾ tsp ginger, grated
- 1 Tbsp hemp seeds, shelled
- 1 ½ tsp turmeric, peeled and grated
- Pinch of cayenne pepper
- 2 or 3 ice cubes

*Directions:*

1. Add solid ingredients then incorporate liquids, blending until smooth. Add ice cubes to increase thickness.
2. Place in the refrigerator until ready to serve.

*Nutrition: 150 calories, 0.5 g saturated fat, 4 g total fat, 25 g carbohydrate, 110 mg sodium, 5.3 g fiber, 5 g protein, 18 g sugar*

***Pineapple Ginger Smoothie***

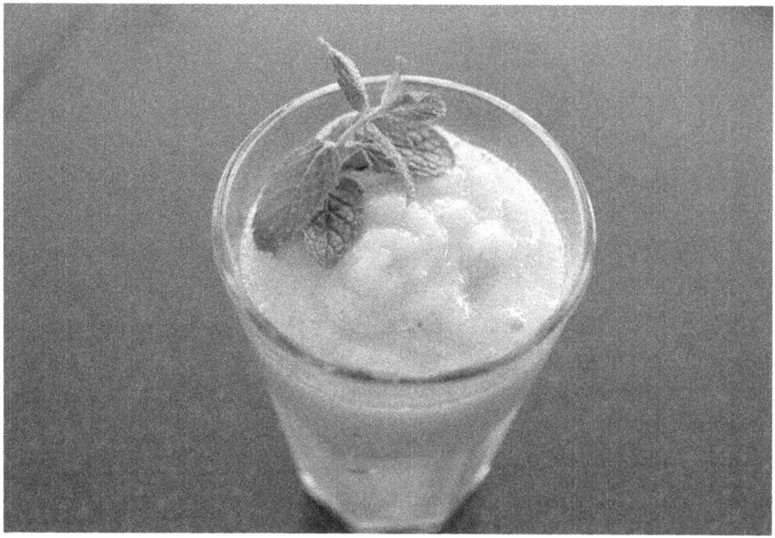

As stated previously, ginger is highly beneficial to your health, and it's loaded with nutrients. Pairing this popular gut-healthy ingredient with pineapple takes to the Bahamas, even if you're stuck at home.

Prep Time: 5 min
Total Time: 5 min
Yield: 2 servings

<u>Ingredients:</u>

- 1 ⅓ cup pineapple chunks, fresh or frozen
- 1 cup unsweetened coconut water
- ½" inch piece ginger, peeled and grated
- ¼ tsp ground turmeric
- 2 or 3 ice cubes

<u>Directions:</u>

1. Add solid ingredients then incorporate liquids, blending until smooth. Add ice cubes to increase thickness.
2. Place in the refrigerator until ready to serve.

<u>Nutrition:</u> *170 calories, 0.2 g saturated fat, 0.5 g total fat, 41 g carbohydrate, 130 mg sodium, 3.2 g fiber, 1.6 g protein, 38 g sugar*

## *Beet and Chia Seed Smoothie*

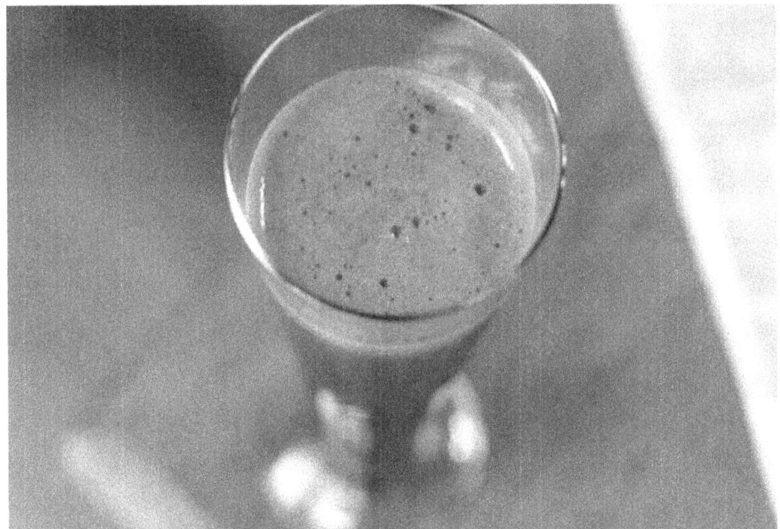

If you've never tried a beet in the past, you've at least likely heard of them from Dwight Schrute's farm. Beets are excellently nutritious and have low-calorie content. Studies conducted on beets have determined that the nitrates absorbed from the beets increase energy in individual cells. They are also noted for improving digestive health. Many people are averse to the taste of beets, but this delicious smoothie will keep you coming back for more.

Prep Time: 5 min
Total Time: 5 min
Yield: 2 servings

*Ingredients:*

- 1 ½ cup unsweetened almond milk
- 1 ½ cup blackberries or blueberries, fresh or frozen
- ½ cup beets, grated
- ½ cup mint leaves
- 4 Tbsp lime juice
- 2 Tbsp chia seeds
- 2 Tbsp honey
- 2 or 3 ice cubes

*Directions:*

1. Add solid ingredients then incorporate liquids, blending until smooth. Add ice cubes to increase thickness.

2.  Place in the refrigerator until ready to serve.

*Nutrition: 320 calories, 1.2 g saturated fat, 12 g total fat, 50 g carbohydrate, 180 mg sodium, 19 g fiber, 8.6 g protein, 26.6 g sugar*

### Honeydew Kiwi Smoothie

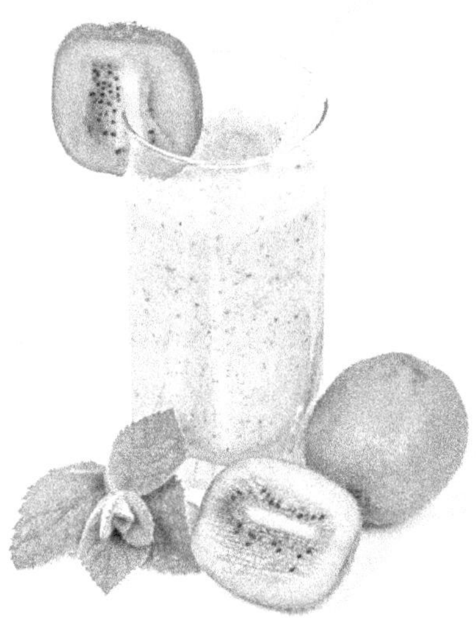

Kiwis are superfruits that are packed with flavor. Kiwis can potentially help children with asthma in children, and they have a lot of fiber, making them perfect for digestion health. Kiwis have also aided in lowering blood pressure and reducing blood clotting, which ultimately improves heart health. With both honeydew and kiwi combined, this smoothie is packed to the brim of healthy ingredients.

Prep Time: 5 min
Total Time: 5 min
Yield: 2 servings

*Ingredients:*

- 2 cups honeydew melon
- 1 ¼ cups kiwi, peeled
- 10 mint leaves
- 1 Tbsp lime juice
- 1 Tbsp honey
- 2 or 3 ice cubes

*Directions:*

1. Add solid ingredients then incorporate liquids, blending until smooth. Add ice cubes to increase thickness.
2. Place in the refrigerator until ready to serve.

*Nutrition: 175 calories, 0.2 g saturated fat, 1 g total fat, 44 g carbohydrate, 45 mg sodium, 6.5 g fiber, 3.2 g protein, 32.4 g sugar*

### Avocado Smoothie

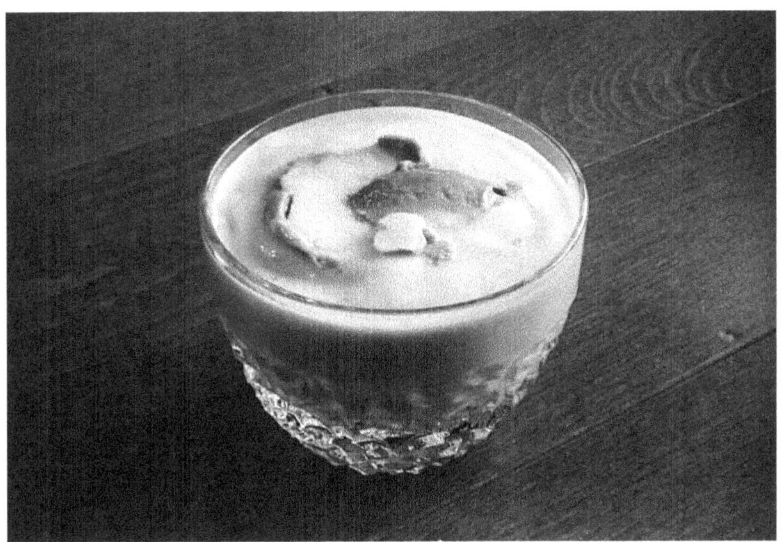

There's a reason that the avocado market has exploded in recent years. Not only are avocados delicious, but they're also incredibly nutritious. Avocados are rich in Vitamins C, E, K, B5, and B6, among other minerals. They're also rich in potassium, containing more than a banana, which is linked to heart and kidney health. If you need a pick-me-up in the form of a smooth fruit, look no further.

Prep Time: 5 min
Total Time: 5 min
Yield: 2 servings

*Ingredients:*

- ½ avocado
- 1 cup coconut water
- 1 tsp agave syrup
- 1 tsp lime juice

*Directions:*

1. Add solid ingredients then incorporate liquids, blending until smooth. Add ice cubes to increase thickness.
2. Place in the refrigerator until ready to serve.

*Nutrition: 140 calories, 2.3 g saturated fat, 10 g total fat, 13.5 g carbohydrate, 130 mg sodium, 5 g fiber, 2 g protein, 3.8 g sugar*

# Chapter 6: Green Smoothies

Green smoothies are all-inclusive meals that capture both fruits and vegetables to give you a balanced diet. Unlike juices, green smoothies are much easier to monitor calorically, and they have fiber that comes from blending whole ingredients. An even blend of fruits and vegetables keeps the calorie amount low while providing excellent nutritional value. Below are some of the best green smoothies to add to your diet.

*Banana Mango Green Smoothie*

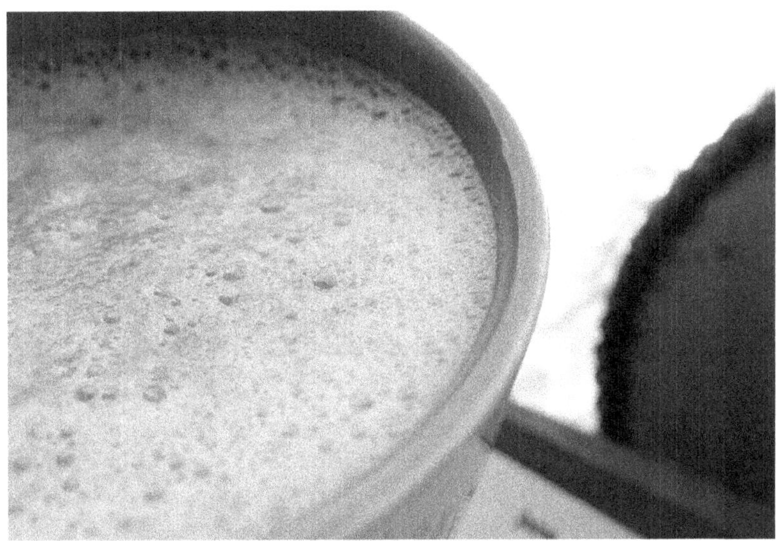

If you're looking for a smoothie that will act as a gateway to your green smoothie journey, this banana mango green smoothie is an excellent place to start. The addition of hemp seeds and kale give this smoothie nutrition packed into a deliciously fruity smoothie.

Prep Time: 5 min
Total Time: 5 min
Yield: 2 servings

*Ingredients:*

- 2 bananas
- 1 cup mangos, fresh or frozen
- 3 handful kale or spinach
- 2 Tbsp hemp seeds

- ½ cup unsweetened almond milk
- 2 or 3 ice cubes

*Directions:*

1. Add solid ingredients then incorporate liquids, blending until smooth. Add ice cubes to increase thickness.
2. Drizzle honey on the top to add to the sweetness.
3. Place in the refrigerator until ready to serve.

*Nutrition: 260 calories, 0.7 g saturated fat, 8.6 g total fat, 42 g carbohydrate, 83 mg sodium, 6 g fiber, 8.5 g protein, 26 g sugar*


## Strawberry Pomegranate Layered Green Smoothie

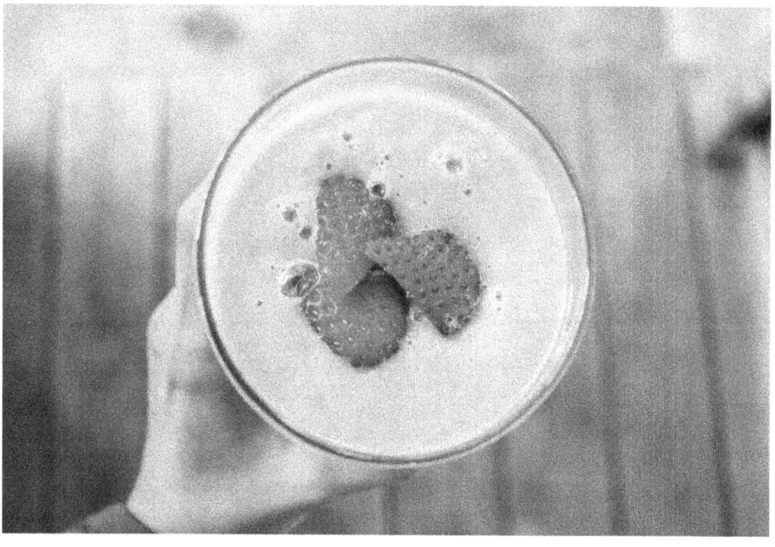

Strawberries and pomegranates make a great pair, and combining them with a layer of green spinach and pomegranate smoothie makes them healthy and fun to eat. You can even add coconut cream to top it off or use coconut milk. Either one will give you a fun, new smoothie experience.

Prep Time: 5 min
Total Time: 5 min
Yield: 2 servings

*Ingredients:*

**Strawberry Pomegranate Layer**

- 1 cup strawberries, fresh or frozen
- 1 banana
- ½ cup coconut water or milk
- 2 or 3 ice cubes

## Spinach Pomegranate Layer

- 1 cup spinach
- ½ banana
- ¼ cup pomegranate arils
- ¼ cup coconut water or milk
- 2 or 3 ice cubes

*Directions:*

1. Add solid ingredients then incorporate liquids, blending until smooth. Add ice cubes to increase thickness.
2. Layer the strawberry pomegranate smoothie on the bottom and the spinach pomegranate smoothie on the top.
3. Place in the refrigerator until ready to serve.

*Nutrition: 200 calories, 1.2 g saturated fat, 2.2 g total fat, 45 g carbohydrate, 56 mg sodium, 4.3 g fiber, 5 g protein, 30 g sugar*


### *Snickerdoodle Green Smoothie*

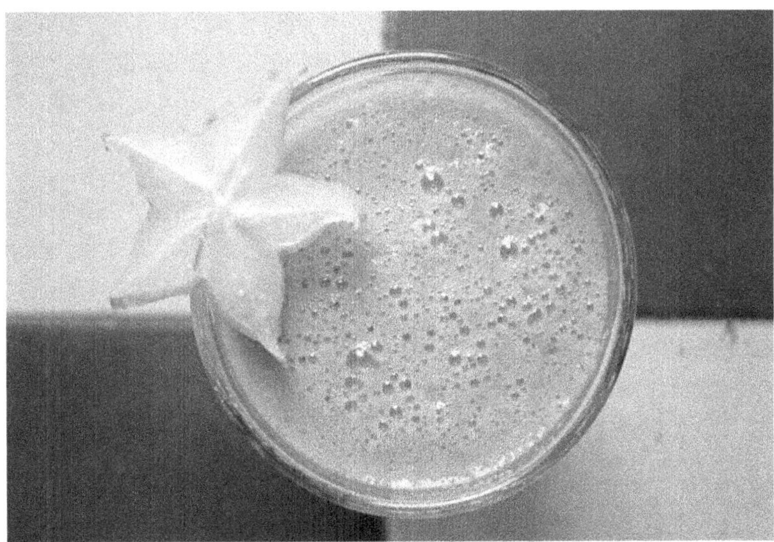

After a long day of work, it's refreshing to know that you'll have something sweet to have at the end of the day. However, if you're trying to lose weight, that can cause a significant problem. This snickerdoodle green smoothie is designed to give you the snickerdoodle taste with the nutritious value of spinach and avocado. Tweak the recipe to give you the right consistency and sweetness.

Prep Time: 5 min
Total Time: 5 min
Yield: 2 servings

*Ingredients:*

- 1 avocado
- 2 bananas
- 2 handfuls of spinach
- ½ cup almond milk
- ½ tsp cinnamon
- 1 tsp vanilla extract
- 2 or 3 ice cubes

*Directions:*

1. Add solid ingredients then incorporate liquids, blending until smooth. Add ice cubes to increase thickness.
2. Place in the refrigerator until ready to serve.

*Nutrients: 335 calories, 4.4 g saturated fat, 21 g total fat, 38 g carbohydrate, 76 mg sodium, 11 g fiber, 4.3 g protein, 15.3 g sugar*

## *Vegan Mango Green Smoothie*

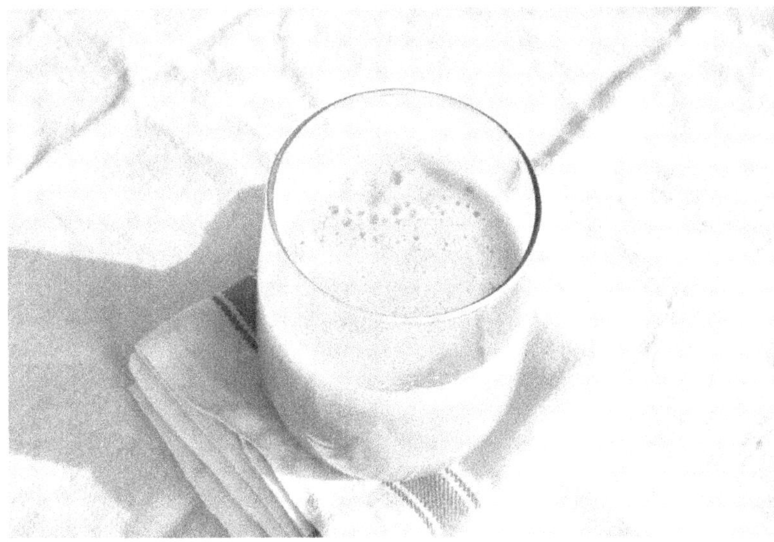

This smoothie is packed with delicious mango and coconut taste that will make you forget about the spinach in it. This heart-healthy morning smoothie is perfect for people looking to start a day with a healthy energy spike. The recipe's only added sugar content is orange juice, but it'll still satisfy your sweet tooth.

Prep Time: 5 min
Total Time: 5 min
Yield: 2 servings

*Ingredients:*

- 1 cup mango, fresh or frozen
- 1 handful spinach
- ½ banana
- ½ cup orange juice
- ¾ cup light coconut milk
- 2 or 3 ice cubes

*Directions:*

1. Add solid ingredients then incorporate liquids, blending until smooth. Add ice cubes to increase thickness.
2. Place in the refrigerator until ready to serve.

*Nutrition: 315 calories, 19 g saturated fat, 22 g total fat, 31 g carbohydrate, 27 mg sodium, 4.5 g fiber, 4 g protein, 23 g sugar*

### *Tropical Green Smoothie*

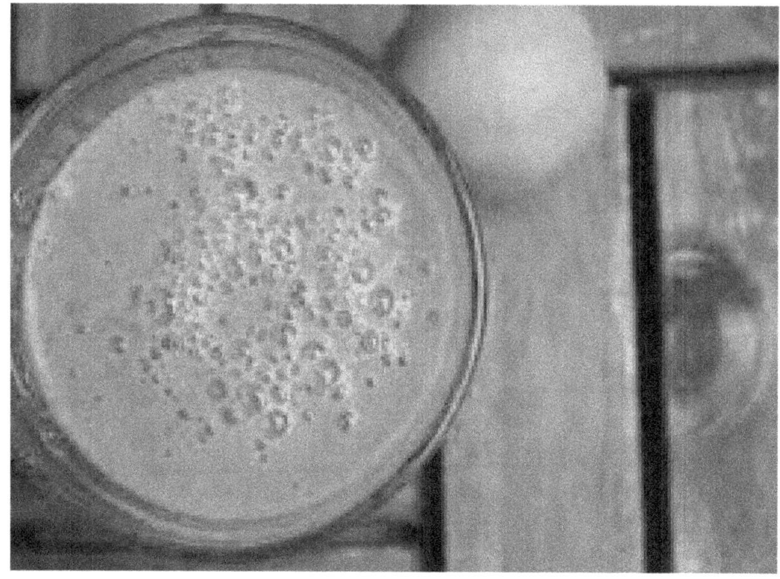

The rich compilation of mango, pineapple, banana, and your favorite berry makes this green smoothie highly customizable and delicious. The addition of spinach gives this smoothie its green color, but you'll likely not notice the taste if you're not a fan of spinach. If you're still looking for more sweetness, add honey, maple syrup, stevia, or sugar.

Prep Time: 5 min
Total Time: 5 min
Yield: 2 servings

*Ingredients:*

- 1 cup pineapple chunks, fresh or frozen
- 1 cup mango chunks, fresh or frozen
- 1 cup strawberries, raspberries, blueberries, or another berry, fresh or frozen
- 1 banana
- 2 cup spinach
- 1 cup unsweetened almond milk
- 1 tsp vanilla extract
- 2 or 3 ice cubes

*Directions:*

1. Add solid ingredients then incorporate liquids, blending until smooth. Add ice cubes to increase thickness.

2. Place in the refrigerator until ready to serve.

*Nutrition:* *300 calories, 1.7 g saturated fat, 3.5 g total fat, 67 g carbohydrate, 86 mg sodium, 6.5 g fiber, 7.2 g protein, 54 g sugar*

### Peanut Butter and Blueberry Smoothie

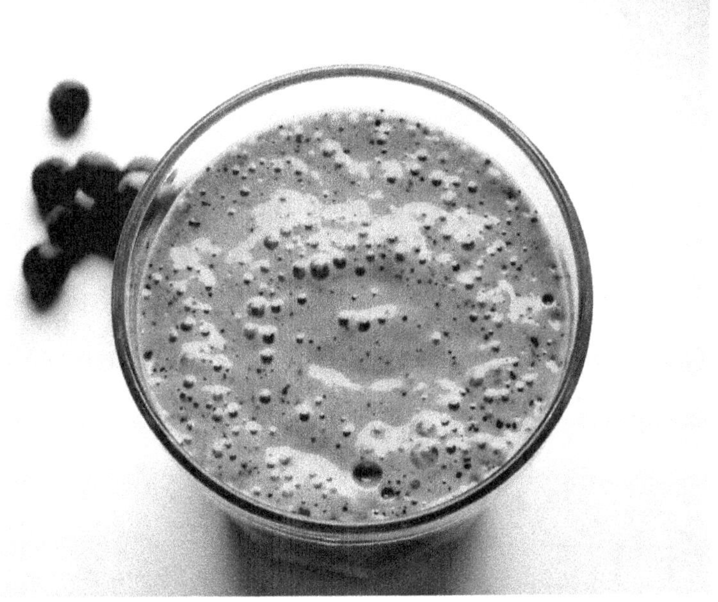

If you're looking for a peanut butter and jelly experience in a smoothie, there's no better place to start than this peanut butter and blueberry smoothie. The rich purple color of this smoothie makes you completely forget that it's also loaded with spinach. If you want to switch it up, consider changing the spinach to kale.

Prep Time: 5 min
Total Time: 5 min
Yield: 2 servings

*Ingredients:*

- 1 cup blueberries
- 1 banana
- 1 handful spinach
- ½ Tbsp peanut butter
- ¼ cup vanilla Greek yogurt
- 1 Tbsp chia seeds
- 2 or 3 ice cubes

*Directions:*

1. Add solid ingredients then incorporate liquids, blending until smooth. Add ice cubes to increase thickness.
2. Place in the refrigerator until ready to serve.

*Nutrition: 280 calories, 1.6 g saturated fat, 12 g total fat, 40 g carbohydrate, 42 mg sodium, 14 g fiber, 9 g protein, 17 g sugar*

## Banana Kale Smoothie

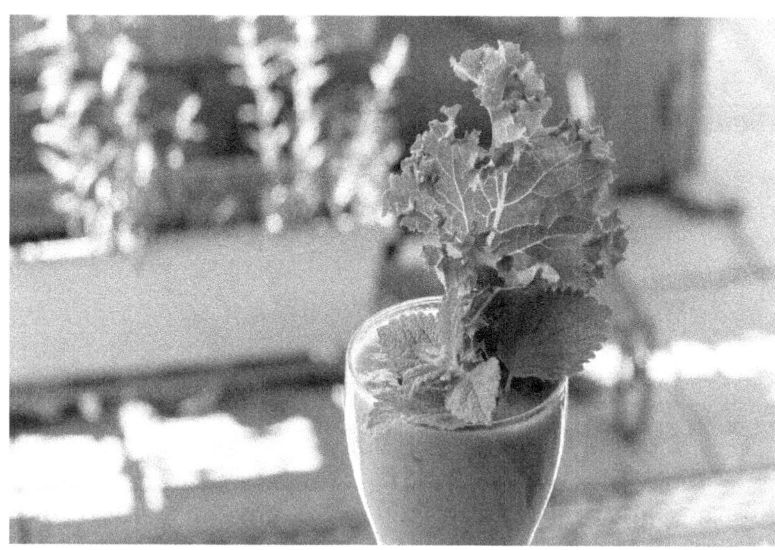

Kale has been a hit for over a decade because it is one of the most nutrient-dense foods out there. It's loaded with vitamins, minerals, and antioxidants that make you feel amazing. Kale is also lauded for helping increase the acids in your stomach to make digestion easier, ultimately lowering cholesterol. Most people don't get their fills of the right vitamins and minerals, but kale is loaded with everything you'll need. So, it's time to start investing in your future and making kale smoothies.

Prep Time: 10 min
Total Time: 10 min
Yield: 2 servings

*Ingredients:*

- 2 bananas
- 1 avocado
- 1 cup kale

- ¼ lemon, juiced
- 2 cups coconut water
- ¼ tsp cayenne pepper
- 2 or 3 ice cubes

*Directions:*

1. Add solid ingredients then incorporate liquids, blending until smooth. Add ice cubes to increase thickness.
2. Place in the refrigerator until ready to serve.

*Nutrition: 375 calories, 5 g saturated fat, 20.5 g total fat, 49 g carbohydrate, 275 mg sodium, 13 g fiber, 6 g protein, 21.4 g sugar*

## Green Detox Smoothie

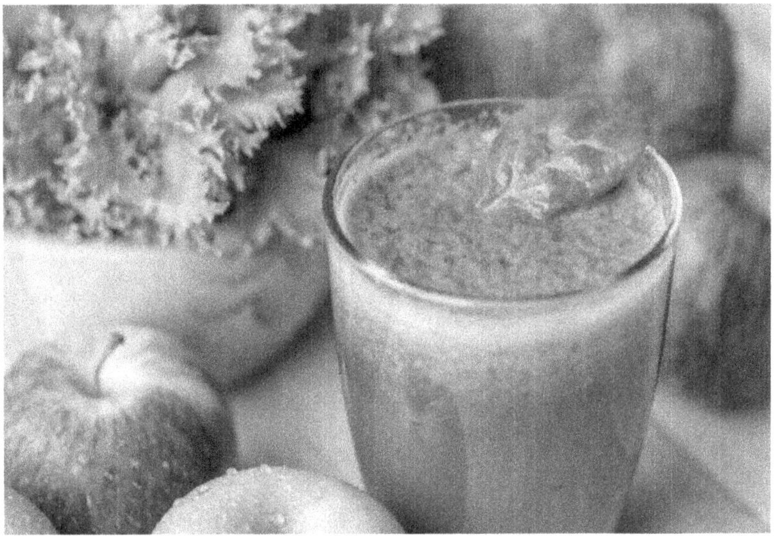

Detoxes are generally ineffective if they are done consistently because, once you return to a regular diet, you gain the weight back. However, occasional detoxes added to your diet may help you lose some weight. If you're on a weight loss journey, consider making this smoothie once a week to start. It's loaded with nutrients and tastes great: a perfect start to your day.

Prep Time: 10 min
Total Time: 10 min
Yield: 2 servings

*Ingredients:*

- ½ pear, chopped
- ½ green apple, chopped
- ½ avocado, chopped
- 1 handful spinach
- ½ cup broccoli florets
- 1 ½ cup pineapple juice
- 2 or 3 ice cubes

*Directions:*

1. Add solid ingredients then incorporate liquids, blending until smooth. Add ice cubes to increase thickness.
2. Place in the refrigerator until ready to serve.

*Nutrition: 380 calories, 1.3 g saturated fat, 9.4 g total fat, 70 g carbohydrate, 170 mg sodium, 18 g fiber, 15 g protein, 34.5 g sugar*


**Berry and Spinach Smoothie**

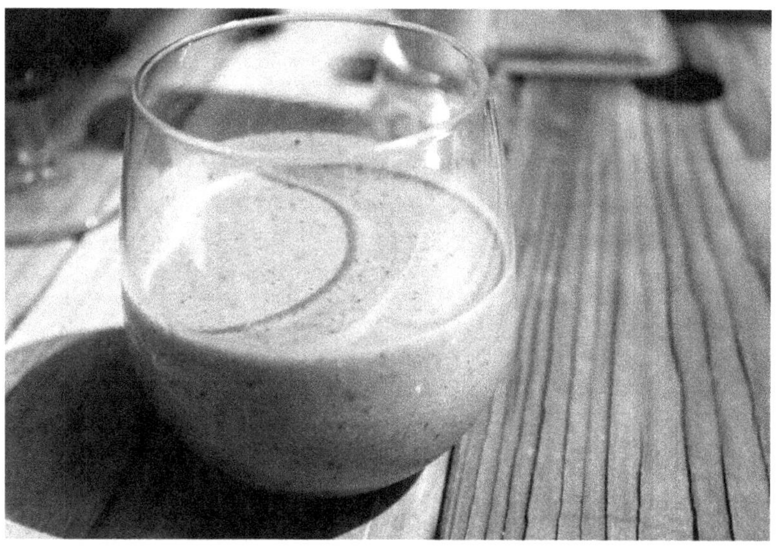

This berry and spinach smoothie also breaks the typical green smoothie mold by giving you a loud pink smoothie. Of course, it completely depends on what you're putting in the smoothie. The berries can range from strawberries to cherries to blackberries, whatever suits you best. Top it off with orange juice, and you've got a beautiful medley to chow down on.

Prep Time: 5 min
Total Time: 5 min

Yield: 2 servings

*Ingredients:*

- 2 cups mixed berries, frozen
- ½ cup strawberries, fresh or frozen
- ¼ cup spinach
- 1 cup vanilla yogurt
- ½ cup orange juice
- 2 or 3 ice cubes

*Directions:*

1. Add solid ingredients then incorporate liquids, blending until smooth. Add ice cubes to increase thickness.
2. Place in the refrigerator until ready to serve.

*Nutrition: 175 calories, 1.2 g saturated fat, 2.6 g total fat, 34.6 g carbohydrate, 90 mg sodium, 4.8 g fiber, 8.2 g protein, 26.4 g sugar*


**Watermelon Green Smoothie**

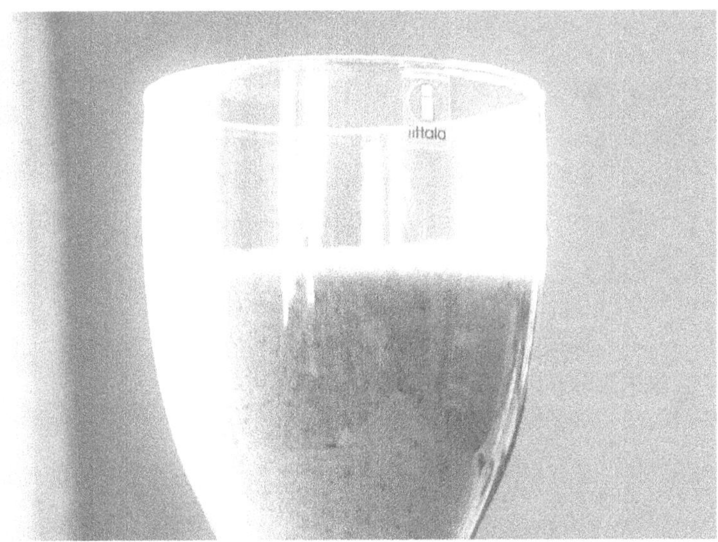


If you've spent the majority of your time trying to find a way to add something other than banana into your smoothie, try this watermelon smoothie. This smoothie contains broccoli, cucumber, celery, and spinach, giving you an excellent assortment of vegetables. At only 65 calories, it's definitely a fan favorite.

Prep Time: 5 min

Total Time: 5 min

Yield: 2 servings

*Ingredients:*

- ½ cup watermelon, diced
- 1 apple, peeled and diced
- 1 cup spinach
- ½ cucumber, sliced
- ½ cup broccoli florets
- 2 stalks celery, chopped
- 2 or 3 ice cubes

*Directions:*

1. Add solid ingredients then incorporate liquids, blending until smooth. Add ice cubes to increase thickness.
2. Place in the refrigerator until ready to serve.

*Nutrition: 65 calories, 0.1 g saturated fat, 0.4 g total fat, 15.3 g carbohydrate, 53.5 mg sodium, 3.5 g fiber, 2 g protein, 9.5 g sugar*


**Ginger Green Smoothie**

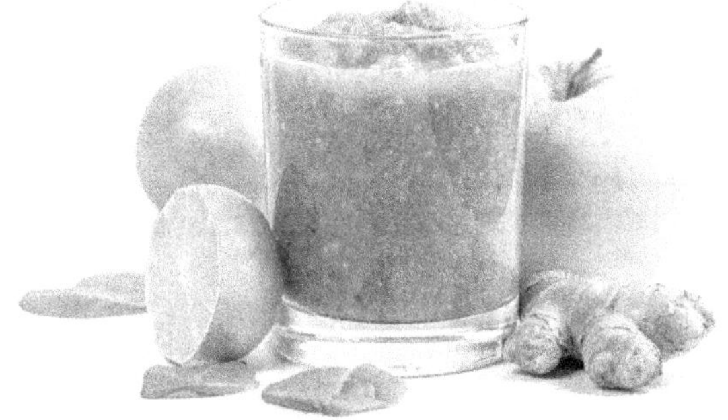

This ginger green smoothie is the perfect wake-up juice before a long day, and it's delicious. It's loaded with vegetables, including kale, ginger, and carrot, and fruits such as avocado and apple. If you're feeling adventurous, add some orange or lime to increase the citrus flavor.

Prep Time: 5 min
Total Time: 5 min
Yield: 2 servings

*Ingredients:*

- 2 avocados
- 2 carrots, chopped
- 2 leaves of kale
- 2 1" pieces of ginger root
- 1 cup parsley
- 2 apples, cored
- 2 lemons, peeled
- 2 Tbsp flax seeds
- ½ cup water
- 2 or 3 ice cubes

*Directions:*

1. Add solid ingredients then incorporate liquids, blending until smooth. Add ice cubes to increase thickness.
2. Place in the refrigerator until ready to serve.

*Nutrition: 530 calories, 5 g saturated fat, 35.7 g total fat, 62.4 g carbohydrate, 106 mg sodium, 28.5 g fiber, 10 g protein, 19 g sugar*

*Banana Peanut Butter Green Smoothie*

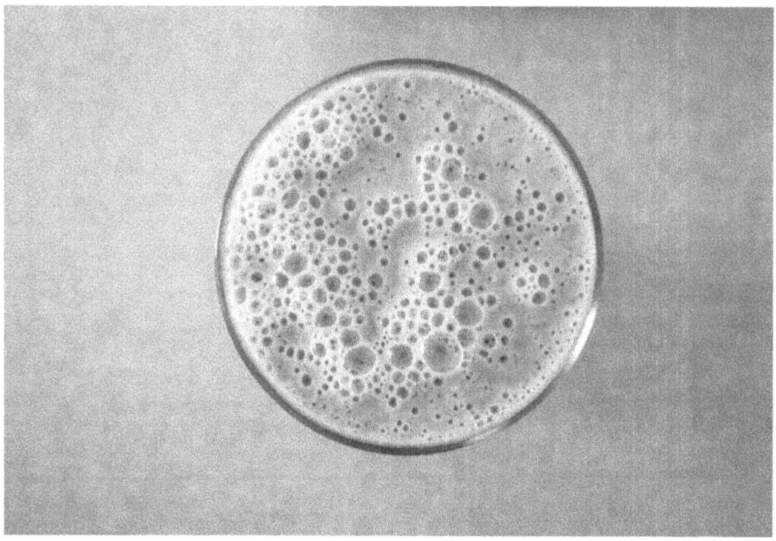

So far, there has been a plethora of breakfast smoothies, but what about the post-workout menu? Well, this smoothie is packed with protein to help you recover after a long workout. This smoothie is also for those new to green smoothies as it only contains spinach.

Prep Time: 5 min
Total Time: 5 min
Yield: 2 servings

*Ingredients:*

- 2 bananas, chopped
- ½ cup spinach
- 2 Tbsp peanut butter
- 1 cup vanilla yogurt
- 2 cup almond milk
- 5 to 10 ice cubes

*Directions:*

1. Add solid ingredients then incorporate liquids, blending until smooth. Add ice cubes to increase thickness.
2. Place in the refrigerator until ready to serve.

*Nutrition: 382 calories, 1.8 g saturated fat, 9.5 g total fat, 55.7 g carbohydrate, 330 mg sodium, 5.4 g fiber, 23.6 g protein, 36 g sugar*

***Orange Banana Green Smoothie***

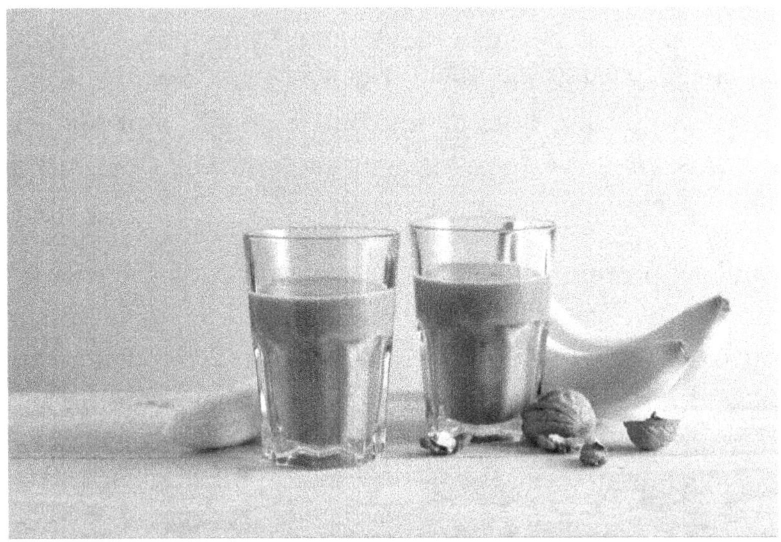

Some say this smoothie tastes like cereal, and it's a great introduction for kids looking to start their green smoothie start. The orange banana green smoothie is low in fat but loaded with vitamin A and fiber. This smoothie is rich and thick, so if you want it runnier, add extra milk. And, best yet, there are only 220 calories!

Prep Time: 5 min
Total Time: 5 min
Yield: 2 servings

*Ingredients:*

- 2 oranges, peeled
- 4 bananas, chopped
- 2 leaves kale
- 1 cup water

*Directions:*

1. Add solid ingredients then incorporate liquids, blending until smooth. Add ice cubes to increase thickness.
2. Place in the refrigerator until ready to serve.

*Nutrition: 220 calories, 0.3 g saturated fat, 1 g total fat, 56 g carbohydrate, 14.5 mg sodium, 6.5 g fiber, 3.2 g protein, 29 g sugar*

# Chapter 7: Protein Smoothies

Protein smoothies are popular because they are great for post-workouts, breakfasts, or even high-protein snacks. There are several ways to get protein from your smoothies, including using protein powder, nuts or nut butter, seeds, and high-protein fruits and vegetables. It's also possible to add protein for your smoothies in unusual places, such as adding garbanzo beans, cottage cheese, or yogurt.

The best way to make a protein shake is to first build your base with frozen fruit or ice. Using frozen fruit will give you a much thicker smoothie, so it's recommended. Next, choose where you want your protein to come from and try using multiple sources of protein in each smoothie. Some protein powders and other protein sources are naturally sweet, but if you need to add more sugar to your smoothie, it's recommended to use natural sweeteners like honey.

### *PB&J Protein Smoothie*

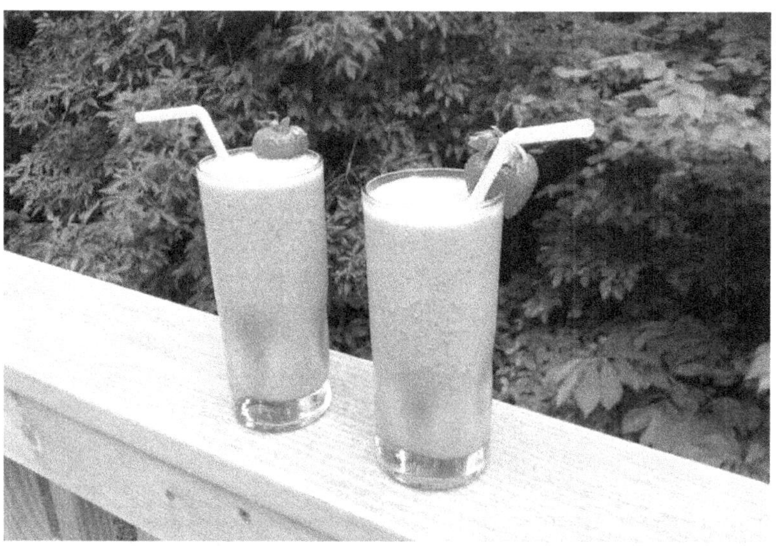

This peanut butter and jelly protein smoothie is perfect for anyone wanting to add a little bit of whimsy with their smoothies. Like most smoothies, this protein smoothie is higher in calories than green or berry smoothies, but it gives you over 34 g of protein in each serving! Experiment with the types of berries you add and even try mixing up the flavors of protein powder.

Prep Time: 5 min

Total Time: 5 min

Yield: 2 servings

<u>*Ingredients:*</u>

- 2 cup mixed berries, fresh or frozen
- 4 Tbsp rolled oats
- 4 Tbsp peanut butter
- ½ cup vanilla protein powder
- 2 cup almond milk
- 2 or 3 ice cubes

<u>*Directions:*</u>

1. Add solid ingredients then incorporate liquids, blending until smooth. Add ice cubes to increase thickness.
2. Place in the refrigerator until ready to serve.

<u>*Nutrition:*</u> *510 calories, 6.6 g saturated fat, 25 g total fat, 43.5 g carbohydrate, 290 mg sodium, 12 g fiber, 34 g protein, 32.3 g sugar*


**Chocolate Coffee Protein Smoothie**

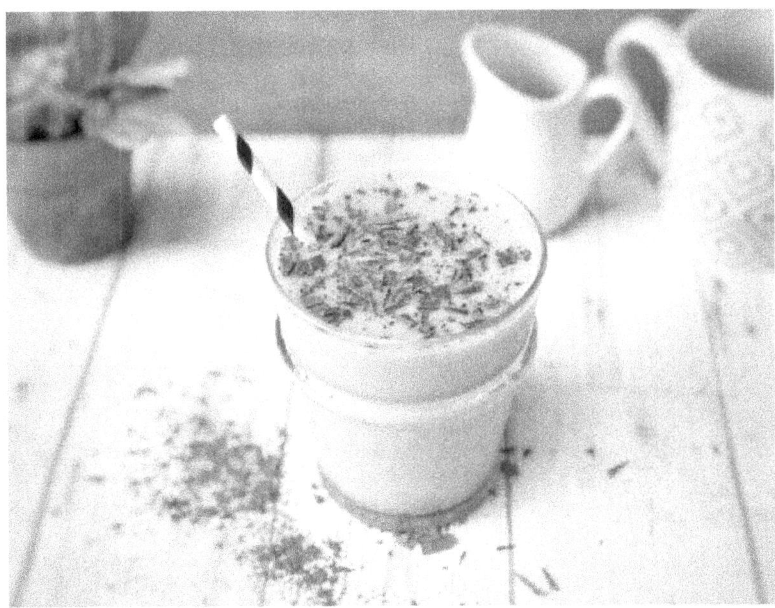

Have you ever craved dessert for breakfast? Well, now you can combine your two favorite parts of the morning: coffee and chocolate. This smoothie contains chocolate protein powder and peanut butter, giving you a creamy morning blend to enhance your caffeine fix. It also comes with the option of cauliflower; maybe it's not your favorite vegetable, but you have to admit that anything you add to this smoothie will make it delicious.

Prep Time: 5 min
Total Time: 5 min
Yield: 2 servings

*Ingredients:*

- 1 banana
- 1 Tbsp natural peanut butter
- ¾ cup cauliflower, frozen
- ½ Tbsp cocoa powder
- 1 scoop chocolate protein powder
- ¼ cup almond milk
- ¾ cup brewed coffee
- 2 or 3 ice cubes

*Directions:*

1. Add solid ingredients then incorporate liquids, blending until smooth. Add ice cubes to increase thickness.
2. Place in the refrigerator until ready to serve.

*Nutrition: 290 calories, 1.5 g saturated fat, 10 g fat, 37.5 g carbohydrates, 50 mg sodium, 9.4 g fiber, 17.7 g protein, 17 g sugar*

*Birthday Cake Protein Smoothie*

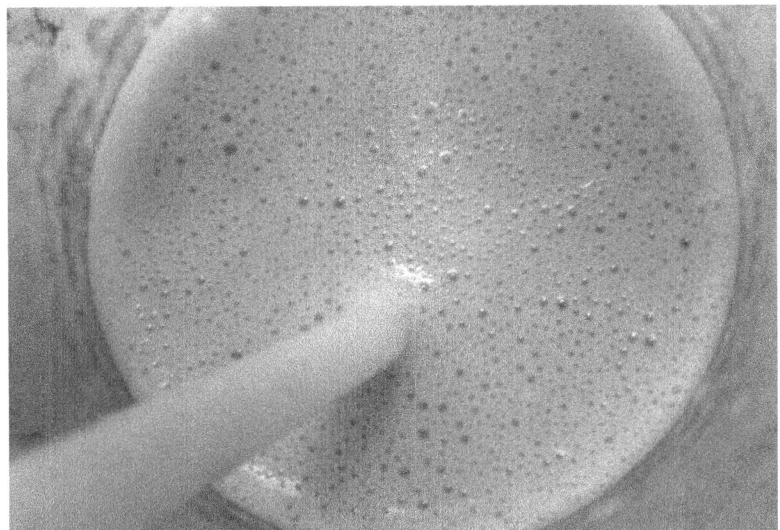

Birthday cake after your workout? Why not! This birthday cake protein smoothie will give you a new outlook when completing your workout. This vanilla cake is perfect for those looking for a sweet alternative to milkshakes while maintaining the whimsy. You can even add sprinkles to spice it up further!

Prep Time: 5 min
Total Time: 5 min
Yield: 2 servings

*Ingredients:*

- 1 large banana
- 2 scoops vanilla protein powder
- ½ cup almond milk
- 1 tsp vanilla
- ½ tsp almond extract
- 1 tsp maple syrup
- 2 or 3 ice cubes

1. Add solid ingredients then incorporate liquids, blending until smooth. Add ice cubes to increase thickness.
2. Place in the refrigerator until ready to serve.

_Nutrition: 325 calories, 13 g saturated fat, 14.6 g total fat, 22 g carbohydrate, 63 mg sodium, 3.6 g fiber, 29 g protein, 13 g sugar_

## Strawberry Protein Smoothie

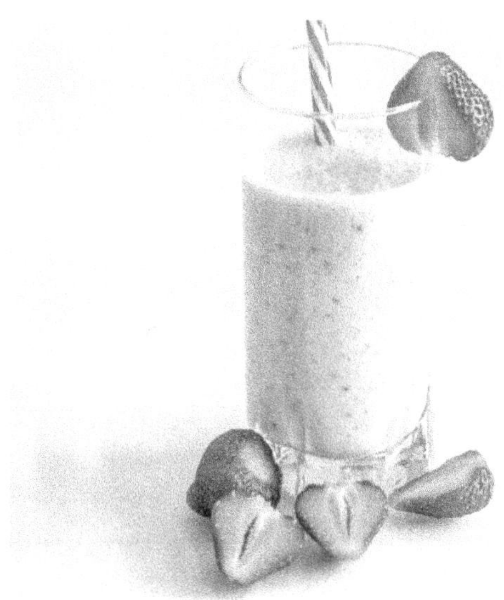

For those of you looking for a way to spice up your already delicious strawberry smoothie, adding protein powder may be your ticket. You can also add graham crackers to the top to add to the crunch. This strawberry protein smoothie will taste more like a trip to the ice cream shop than it will a nutritious meal.

Prep Time: 5 min
Total Time: 5 min
Yield: 2 servings

_Ingredients:_

- 1 ½ cup strawberries, fresh or frozen
- ½ banana
- ⅓ cup vanilla Greek yogurt
- 1 scoop vanilla protein powder
- 1 cup unsweetened almond milk

- 2 or 3 ice cubes



*Directions:*

1. Add solid ingredients then incorporate liquids, blending until smooth. Add ice cubes to increase thickness.
2. Place in the refrigerator until ready to serve.

*Nutrition: 170 calories, 0.5 g saturated fat, 2.8 g total fat, 21 g carbohydrate, 125 mg sodium, 4 g fiber, 17.5 g protein, 12.7 g sugar*

## Banana Protein Smoothie

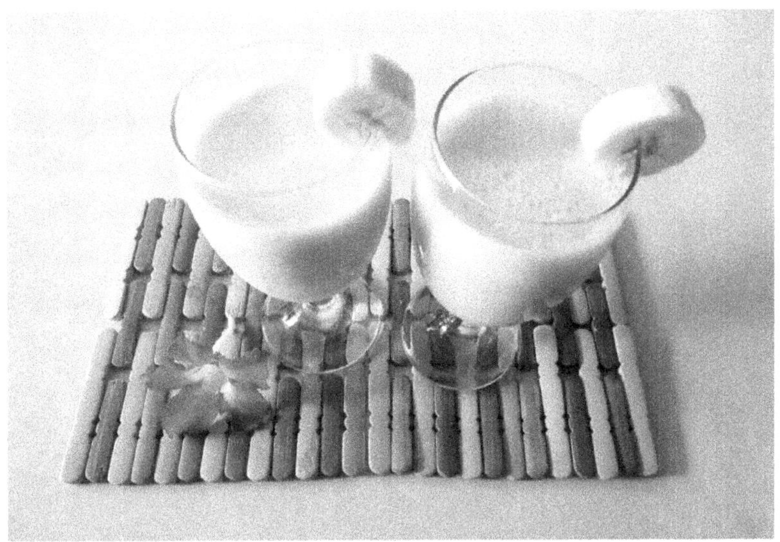

It would be remiss to add a protein smoothie section without adding banana, one of the top fruits listed. This smoothie contains 16 g of protein and gets its creaminess from the delicious banana. You can eat this as an after-workout recovery smoothie or as a breakfast pick-me-up. Either way, this smoothie, which only contains 180 calories, will have you repeatedly coming back for more.

Prep Time: 5 min
Total Time: 5 min
Yield: 2 servings

*Ingredients:*

- 1 banana
- ½ cup vanilla Greek yogurt
- 1 scoop vanilla protein powder

- 1 cup unsweetened almond milk
- 1 tsp vanilla extract
- 2 or 3 ice cubes

*Directions:*

1. Add solid ingredients then incorporate liquids, blending until smooth. Add ice cubes to increase thickness.
2. Place in the refrigerator until ready to serve.

*Nutrition: 180 calories, 0.6 g saturated fat, 2.7 g total fat, 20.5 g carbohydrate, 130 mg sodium, 2.3 g fiber, 18 g protein, 12 g sugar*


**Superfood Protein Smoothie**

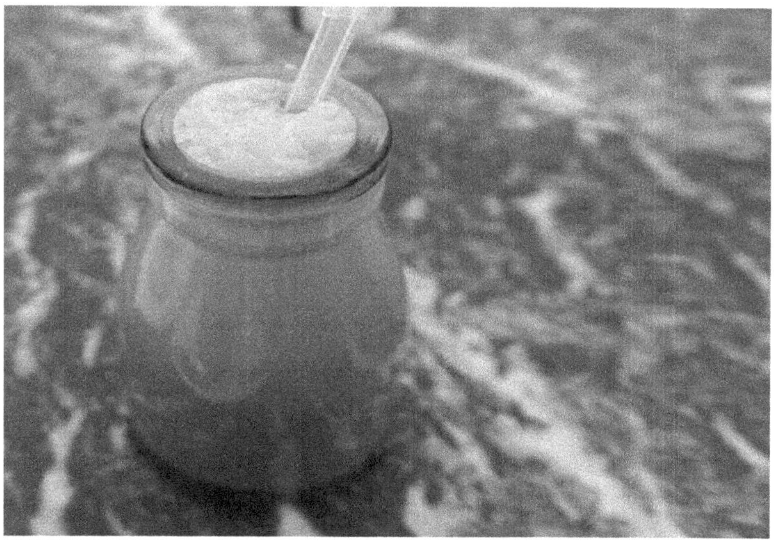

This protein smoothie has it all. If you wanted a green, protein-packed smoothie, this should be your first stop. Though you can use any type of protein powder, it's recommended that you use chocolate to accent the cocoa powder. This creamy smoothie is naturally sweetened with Medjool dates, a healthy alternative to sugar.

Prep Time: 5 min
Total Time: 5 min
Yield: 2 servings

*Ingredients:*

- 1 banana
- 1 cup blueberries, fresh or frozen

- 2 Medjool dates, pitted
- 1 cup kale
- ½ cup cauliflower florets, frozen
- ½ Tbsp flaxseed, ground
- 1 ½ Tbsp cocoa powder
- 2 cup chocolate protein powder
- 2 cups unsweetened almond milk
- 2 or 3 ice cubes

*Directions:*

1. Add solid ingredients then incorporate liquids, blending until smooth. Add ice cubes to increase thickness.
2. Place in the refrigerator until ready to serve.

*Nutrition: 365 calories, 1.8 g saturated fat, 6.6 g total fat, 58.5 g carbohydrate, 365 mg sodium, 10 g fiber, 25.7 g protein, 35 g sugar*

### Date and Dark Chocolate Protein Smoothie

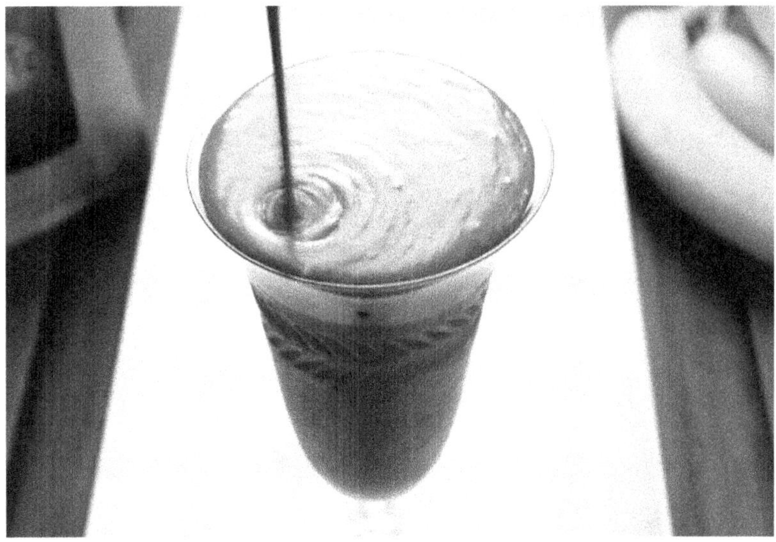

In case you've never had the pleasure of trying dates and dark chocolate, here's your chance. The dates give a caramel flavor and, paired with dark chocolate, you'll think you're eating a candy bar. This protein smoothie only has 42 g of sugar, far below what you'd expect from a smoothie of this caliber. Of course, if you're feeling confident about adding more sugar, consider changing the milk to chocolate milk for kicks and giggles.

Prep Time: 5 min

Total Time: 5 min
Yield: 2 servings

*Ingredients:*

- 2 bananas
- 3 Medjool dates, pitted
- 1 cup kale
- 3 Tbsp dark cocoa powder
- ½ tsp vanilla extract
- 1 cup unsweetened almond milk
- 2 or 3 ice cubes

*Directions:*

1. Add solid ingredients then incorporate liquids, blending until smooth. Add ice cubes to increase thickness.
2. Place in the refrigerator until ready to serve.

*Nutrition:* 280 calories, 0.3 g saturated fat, 3 g total fat, 67.6 g carbohydrate, 200 mg sodium, 10 g fiber, 6 g protein, 42 g sugar


**Peppermint Dark Chocolate Protein Smoothie**

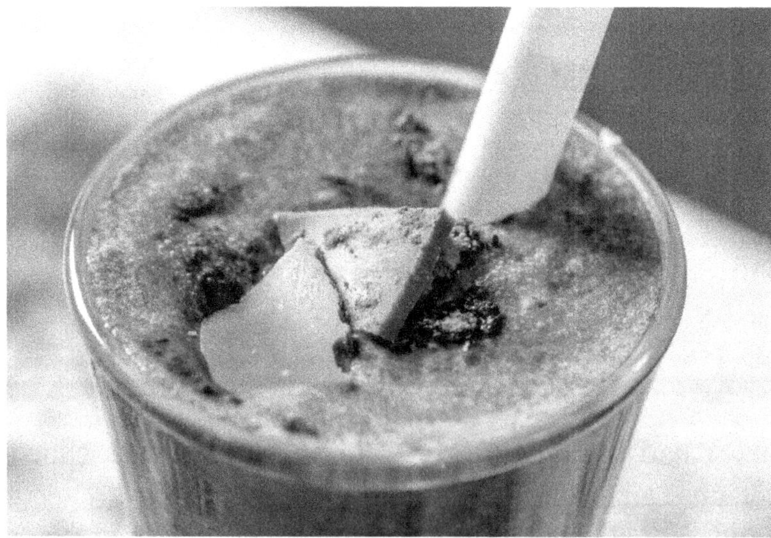

Peppermint is often associated with Christmas, but you can truly enjoy this peppermint dark chocolate protein smoothie anytime. Consider using this smoothie as a treat for

yourself after a long workout or after a long day of work. If you want to make it even more decadent, you can add some dark chocolate shavings and whipped cream.

Prep Time: 5 min
Total Time: 5 min
Yield: 2 servings

*Ingredients:*

- 2 large bananas
- 4 Tbsp cocoa powder
- 2 cup unsweetened almond milk
- 2 scoop chocolate protein powder
- ½ tsp peppermint extract
- 2 or 3 ice cubes

*Directions:*

1. Add solid ingredients then incorporate liquids, blending until smooth. Add ice cubes to increase thickness.
2. Place in the refrigerator until ready to serve.

*Nutrition: 245 calories, 1.8 g saturated fat, 6 g total fat, 41 g carbohydrate, 265 mg sodium, 8 g fiber, 14.4 g protein, 18 g sugar*


### Cherry Chocolate Smoothie

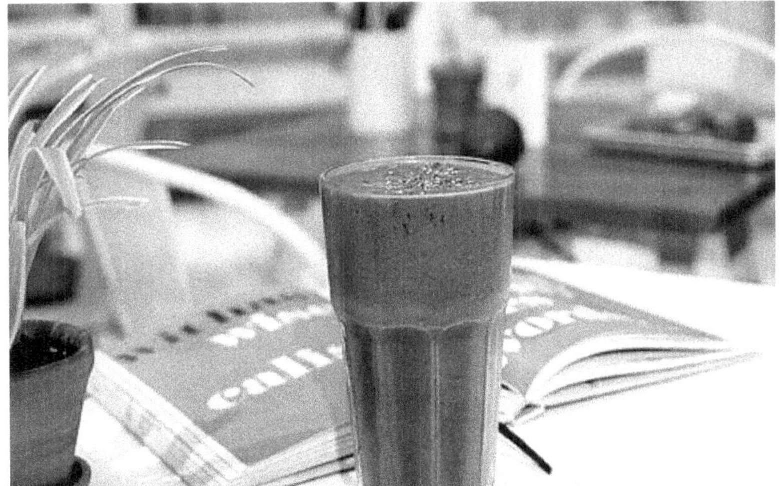

Cherries are highly effective in relieving soreness, so what better time to take a cherry chocolate smoothie than after a workout. This smoothie contains both fruits and vegetables finished with walnuts and flax seeds. Though the smoothie is higher in calories than the others, you'll likely get a better return on your recovery.

Prep Time: 5 min
Total Time: 5 min
Yield: 2 servings

*Ingredients:*

- 2 cups dark cherries, pitted
- 1 cup spinach
- 2 scoops chocolate protein powder
- 1 Tbsp walnuts
- 1 Tbsp ground flax
- 1 Tbsp dark cocoa powder
- 1 ½ cup unsweetened almond milk
- 2 or 3 ice cubes

*Directions:*

1. Add solid ingredients then incorporate liquids, blending until smooth. Add ice cubes to increase thickness.
2. Place in the refrigerator until ready to serve.

*Nutrition: 300 calories, 1.3 g saturated fat, 9.3 g total fat, 46 g carbohydrate, 260 mg sodium, 9.7 g fiber, 17.3 g protein, 27 g sugar*

*Pumpkin Vanilla Protein Smoothie*

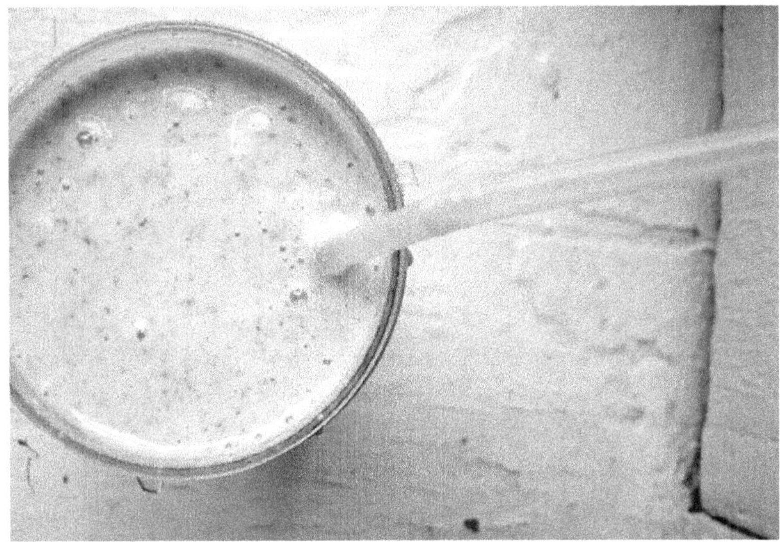

Just like most of these protein smoothies, you can get away with some of the best flavors when you combine them with protein powder. This smoothie tastes like a pumpkin pie, and it's also good for your skin and eyes, packing a punch of vitamin A. Try adding cinnamon sprinkled on top to get more of that pie taste.

Prep Time: 5 min
Total Time: 5 min
Yield: 2 servings

<u>Ingredients:</u>

- ¾ cup pureed pumpkin
- 2 scoops vanilla protein powder
- ½ cup uncooked oats
- 1 ½ cup unsweetened almond milk
- 1 Tbsp walnuts
- 1 Tbsp ground flax
- 1 tsp vanilla extract
- 2 or 3 ice cubes

<u>Directions:</u>

1. Add solid ingredients then incorporate liquids, blending until smooth. Add ice cubes to increase thickness.
2. Place in the refrigerator until ready to serve.

*Nutrition:* *300 calories, 1 g saturated fat, 8.6 g total fat, 22.6 g carbohydrate, 193 mg sodium, 6.7 g fiber, 33.6 g protein, 2.3 g sugar*

**Double Chocolate Mint Smoothie**

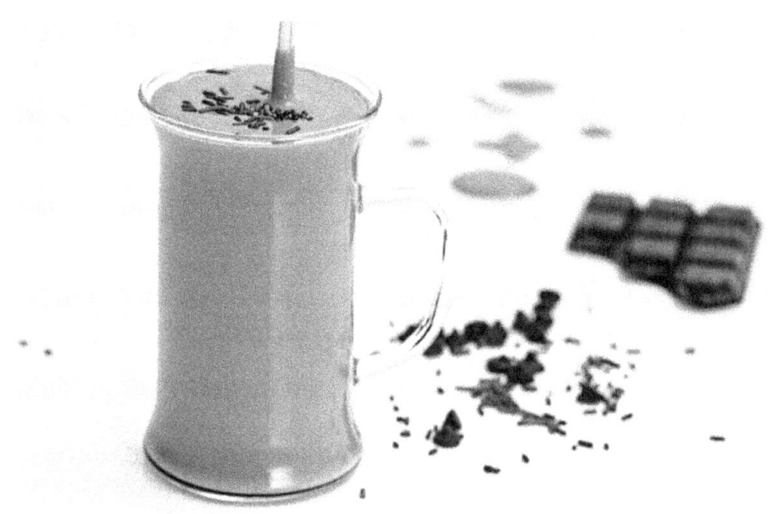

Are you obsessed with chocolate mint flavoring? Well, now you have an excuse to dive into a double chocolate mint smoothie that will have you feeling refreshed. This smoothie contains chocolate protein powder, chocolate almond milk, chocolate powder, and chocolate chips; everything you'd want in a smoothie. Best, yet, it's high in protein and low in calories.

Prep Time: 5 min
Total Time: 5 min
Yield: 2 servings

*Ingredients:*

- 1 scoop chocolate protein powder
- 2 Tbsp unsweetened cocoa powder
- 1 Tbsp chocolate chips
- ¾ cup chocolate almond milk
- ¼ cup water
- 1 Tbsp walnuts
- 2 mint leaves
- 2 or 3 ice cubes

*Directions:*

1. Add solid ingredients then incorporate liquids, blending until smooth. Add ice cubes to increase thickness.
2. Place in the refrigerator until ready to serve.

*Nutrition: 150 calories, 2 g saturated fat, 6.2 g total fat, 16.7 g carbohydrate, 106 mg sodium, 3.6 g fiber, 8.2 g protein, 11 g sugar*

### Coconut Almond Smoothie

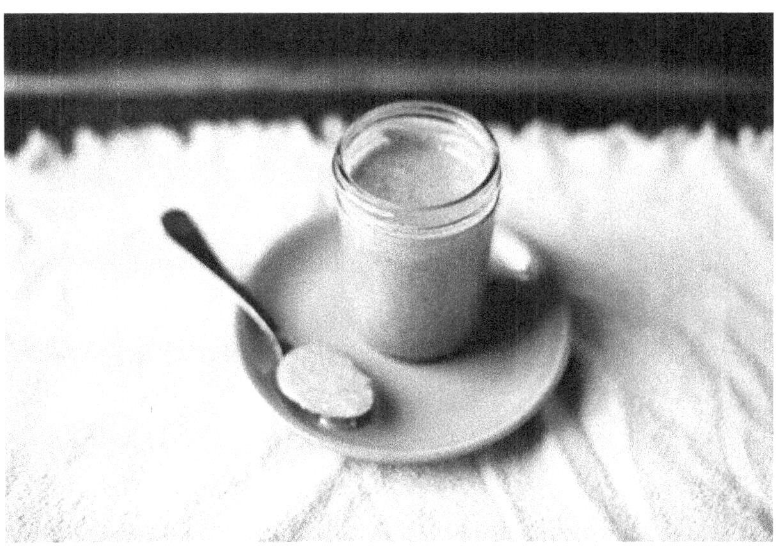

This white decadent chocolate smoothie is packed with unsweetened coconut and almond. This smoothie is for those who like thick, creamy smoothies, and you can even add whipped cream to the top.

Prep Time: 5 min
Total Time: 5 min
Yield: 2 servings

*Ingredients:*

- 1 Tbsp almond butter
- 1 scoop chocolate protein powder
- 1 Tbsp coconut flakes
- 1 cup chocolate almond milk
- 1 ½ cup water
- 2 or 3 ice cubes

*Directions:*

1. Add solid ingredients then incorporate liquids, blending until smooth. Add ice cubes to increase thickness.
2. Place in the refrigerator until ready to serve.

*Nutrition:* *150 calories, 1.1 g saturated fat, 6.6 g total fat, 3.4 g carbohydrate, 135 mg sodium, 1.5 g fiber, 16 g protein, 0.5 g sugar*

### Blueberry Breakfast Smoothies

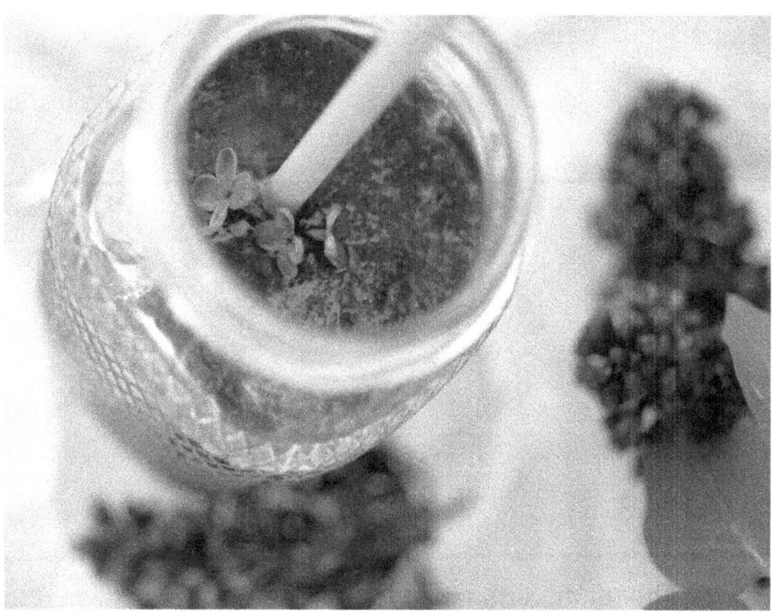

This breakfast smoothie can be eaten as either a drink or a bowl, but a bowl is more fun. The walnuts, oats, and chia seeds can be placed on the top of the smoothie, and consider adding blueberries and banana slices to make the smoothie extra bowl-friendly. This protein-packed smoothie is the perfect way to start your day.

Prep Time: 5 min
Total Time: 5 min
Yield: 2 servings

*Ingredients:*

- 1 cup blueberries
- ½ banana
- 1 ½ scoops protein powder
- 2 Tbsp oats
- 2 Tbsp walnuts

- 1 Tbsp chia seeds
- 2 or 3 ice cubes

<u>Directions:</u>

1. Add solid ingredients then incorporate liquids, blending until smooth. Add ice cubes to increase thickness.
2. Place in the refrigerator until ready to serve.

<u>Nutrition:</u> *365 calories, 2 g saturated fat, 15.5 g total fat, 36.2 g carbohydrate, 47 mg sodium, 13.3 fiber, 25 g protein, 11.6 g sugar*

## Matcha Smoothie

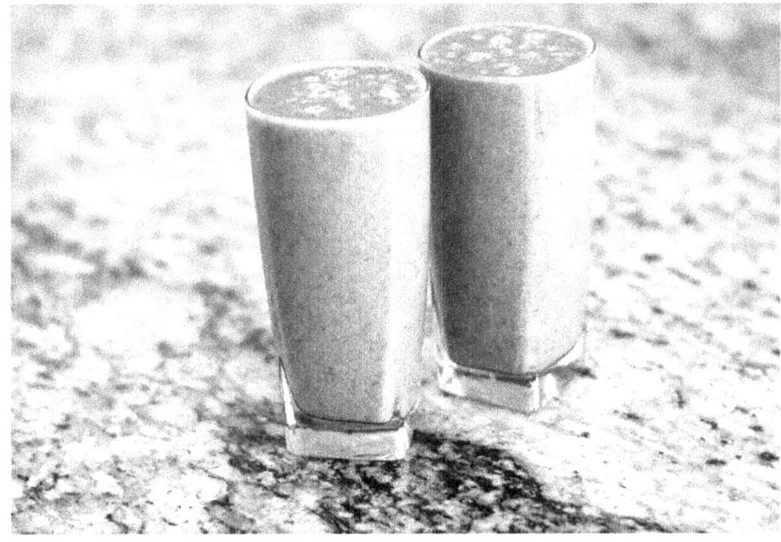

Matcha tea has become extremely popular over the last few years, and it's extremely healthy. Matcha is high in antioxidants that help repair damaged cells. Matcha tea is also used to aid liver problems and may prevent liver diseases in the future. It's also responsible for boosting brain power, which puts it at the top of the list for the perfect breakfast smoothie.

Prep Time: 5 min
Total Time: 5 min
Yield: 2 servings

<u>Ingredients:</u>

- 1 cup mango, fresh or frozen
- 1 tsp matcha tea powder

- 1 Tbsp cashew butter
- 2 scoops vanilla protein powder
- 1 Tbsp lime juice
- 1 cup coconut milk
- ¼ tsp ginger powder
- 2 or 3 ice cubes

*Directions:*

1. Add solid ingredients then incorporate liquids, blending until smooth. Add ice cubes to increase thickness.
2. Place in the refrigerator until ready to serve.

*Nutrition: 500 calories, 26.3 g saturated fat, 33 g total fat, 23.7 g carbohydrate, 74 mg sodium, 5.3 g fiber, 32.5 g protein, 16 g sugar*

# Conclusion

If you feel lost and are unsure on what to do to improve your health, you're not alone. Millions of people suffer from health problems, dull skin, lack of energy, and weight gain, and many of those forget to take the time to improve their lives. The smoothies in this book are designed to give you a quick alternative to healthy foods that will not take a lot of time or money. After all, your health shouldn't have to cost you a fortune.

Smoothies have been proven to aid in weight loss when paired with exercise and a good diet. Smoothies increase your energy levels and improve health issues you may not have known that you have. Most people eat smoothies for breakfast because they like to have a boost of energy early in the morning. In fact, if you are converting to eating smoothies for breakfast, you may even see a higher level of energy than drinking down several glasses of coffee. Smoothies are responsible for giving you glowing skin and improving acne—if you use the right ingredients. If you know what you're looking for, you can pack any nutrients into your smoothie, making it healthier than ever.

While most nutritionists say that eating fruit whole is better for you than a smoothie, as long as your smoothies are thick, you will get the same benefits. However, many people make mistakes when they make their smoothies: Having a glass too large packs in more calories; a smoothie with too many ingredients can overpower the flavors of the smoothie and the nutrients; eating smoothies from take-out locations usually involves eating a lot of sugar; not eating a smoothie with a spoon will not fill you up as quickly, and drinking a smoothie at the wrong time of day won't give you all the health benefits you want. So, before you start drinking smoothies full-time, lay out a schedule for success.

When making your smoothies, choose fruit that will give you the right balance of nutrients that will keep you full for the rest of the day. When adding liquid, don't forget to include creamy liquids, such as almond or coconut milk, to give you an extra burst of flavor and to ultimately thicken the smoothie. If you're feeling adventurous, invest in add-ins, such as granola or almonds. Finally, add ice to the mixture to thicken your smoothie and give it a nice chill.

If you're new to smoothies, you've likely mostly heard of fruit and vegetable smoothies, and for good reason: They're healthy and give you lots of flavor. Berry smoothies are also fan favorites, and diving into different types of berries can increase the likelihood of finding health benefits. Unusual berries, such as boysenberries or elderberries, are great additions and are filled with antioxidants.

Dive into a wide array of combo smoothies that give you perks you may not have considered. For example, adding CBD oil to your smoothie may lower your pain levels. Green smoothies are all the rage, so it's time you found some that you can list in your favorites list. Finally, protein smoothies give you energy to start the day and to recover after a workout.

If there's one thing to remember, it's to always experiment with your smoothies. Getting healthier is sometimes an uncomfortable journey, but that doesn't mean you have to suffer through foods you hate. Find what you love and build around your favorite recipes to give yourself as many options as possible.

# Leave the review

If you enjoyed this book, I'd really appreciate it if you left your honest feedback. I love hearing from my readers and I personally read every single review.

# References

A Couple Cooks. (2020a, June 17). *Easy Beet Smoothie*. A Couple Cooks.
    https://www.acouplecooks.com/beet-smoothie/

A Couple Cooks. (2020b, August 21). *Magic Broccoli Smoothie*. A Couple Cooks.
    https://www.acouplecooks.com/broccoli-smoothie/

A Couple Cooks. (2020c, September 15). *Perfect Carrot Smoothie*. A Couple Cooks.
    https://www.acouplecooks.com/carrot-smoothie/

A Couple Cooks. (2020d, September 30). *Creamy Pumpkin Smoothie*. A Couple Cooks.
    https://www.acouplecooks.com/pumpkin-smoothie/

A Spicy Perspective. (2020, April 8). *Simple Strawberry Smoothie Recipe*. A Spicy Perspective.
    https://www.aspicyperspective.com/simple-strawberry-smoothies/

Allrecipes. (2019). *Blueberry Smoothie Recipe*. Allrecipes.
    https://www.allrecipes.com/recipe/215184/blueberry-smoothie/

Allrecipes. (n.d.-a). *Green Detox Smoothie*. Allrecipes.
    https://www.allrecipes.com/recipe/238998/green-detox-smoothie/

Allrecipes. (n.d.-b). *Green Monster Smoothie.*Allrecipes.
    https://www.allrecipes.com/recipe/222708/green-monster-smoothie/

Allrecipes. (n.d.-c). *Healthy Berry and Spinach Smoothie*. Allrecipes.
    https://www.allrecipes.com/recipe/240726/healthy-berry-and-spinach-smoothie/

Allrecipes. (n.d.-d). *Jumping Ginger Smoothie*. Allrecipes.
    https://www.allrecipes.com/recipe/231321/jumping-ginger-smoothie/

Allrecipes. (n.d.-e). *Kale Banana Smoothie*. Allrecipes.
    https://www.allrecipes.com/recipe/237136/kale-banana-smoothie/

Allrecipes. (n.d.-f). *Kale Orange Banana Smoothie*. Allrecipes.
    https://www.allrecipes.com/recipe/220172/kale-orange-banana-smoothie/

Allrecipes. (n.d.-g). *Watermelon Refreshing Green Smoothie*. Allrecipes.
    https://www.allrecipes.com/recipe/260168/watermelon-refreshing-green-smoothie/

Ambition Kitchen. (2019, July 11). *Good Morning Coffee Smoothie*. Ambitious Kitchen.
    https://www.ambitiouskitchen.com/good-morning-coffee-smoothie/

Ball, J. (2020, January 20). *Health Benefits of Turmeric & Ginger*. EatingWell.
    https://www.eatingwell.com/article/7561449/health-benefits-of-turmeric-ginger/

Baraghani, A. (2017, April 26). *Roasted Strawberry and Tahini Buttermilk Shake*. Bon Appétit.
    https://www.bonappetit.com/recipe/roasted-strawberry-and-tahini-buttermilk-shake

Baraghani, A. (2019, April 29). *CBD Mango Smoothie*. Bon Appétit.
    https://www.bonappetit.com/recipe/cbd-mango-smoothie

Baz, M. (2018a, June 20). *Chill-Out Honeydew Cucumber Slushy Recipe*. Bon Appetit.
    https://www.bonappetit.com/recipe/chill-out-honeydew-cucumber-slushy

Baz, M. (2018b, June 20). *Inflammation-Busting Pineapple Slushy*. Bon Appétit. https://www.bonappetit.com/recipe/inflammation-busting-pineapple-slushy

Bjarnadottir, A. (2019, February 22). *Mulberries 101: Nutrition Facts and Health Benefits*. Healthline. https://www.healthline.com/nutrition/foods/mulberries#vitamins-and-minerals

Bon Appetit Test Kitchen. (2010, May 17). *Honeydew-Kiwi Smoothie*. Bon Appétit. https://www.bonappetit.com/recipe/honeydew-kiwi-smoothie

Brown, M. J. (2017, June 15). *Fresh vs Frozen Fruit and Vegetables — Which Are Healthier?* Healthline. https://www.healthline.com/nutrition/fresh-vs-frozen-fruit-and-vegetables#TOC_TITLE_HDR_3

Butler, N. (2014, November 25). *Kiwi Benefits: Asthma, Digestion, Vision Loss, and More*. Healthline. https://www.healthline.com/health/7-best-things-about-kiwi#protects-against-vision-loss

Butler, N. (2017, December 21). *Nutrition: Great Foods for Getting Vitamins A to K in Your Diet*. Healthline. https://www.healthline.com/health/foods-nutrition-vitamins-a-b-c-d-e-k#vitamin-a

Castellano, S. (2017, March 27). *Green Smoothie Bowls with Mango + Hemp Seeds*. With Food And Love. https://withfoodandlove.com/banana-mango-green-smoothie-bowls-with-hemp-seeds-sprouts-vegan/

Coyle, D. (2017, May 26). *9 Impressive Health Benefits of Beets*. Healthline. https://www.healthline.com/nutrition/benefits-of-beets#TOC_TITLE_HDR_6

Cronkleton, E. (2017, May 5). *Wheatgrass: Benefits, Side Effects, and More*. Healthline. https://www.healthline.com/health/food-nutrition/wheatgrass-benefits#immune-system

Danahy, A. (2019, July 23). *5 Health and Nutrition Benefits of Coconut*. Healthline. https://www.healthline.com/nutrition/coconut-nutrition#TOC_TITLE_HDR_5

Daou, A. (2017, May 2). *Mulberry morning smoothie*. Anna's cooking concept. https://annacookingconcept.com/mulberry-morning-smoothie/

Delish Knowledge. (2018, December 26). *Healing Cranberry Smoothie*. Delish Knowledge. https://www.delishknowledge.com/healing-cranberry-smoothie/#tasty-recipes-20913-jump-target

Dinner at the Zoo. (2017, January 9). *Mixed Berry Smoothie*. Dinner at the Zoo. https://www.dinneratthezoo.com/mixed-berry-smoothie/

Dinner at the Zoo. (2018, February 19). *Raspberry Smoothie*. Dinner at the Zoo. https://www.dinneratthezoo.com/raspberry-smoothie/#wprm-recipe-container-12073

Eaves, A., Kadey, M., & Matthews, M. (2020, August 13). *22 High-Protein Smoothies That Actually Keep You Full*. Men's Health. https://www.menshealth.com/nutrition/a19545933/healthy-protein-smoothie-recipes/

Ferreira, M., & Ayuda, T. (2019, December 27). *5 Ways Your Smoothie Is Making You Gain Weight—And How to Fix It*. Prevention. https://www.prevention.com/weight-loss/g20430598/smoothie-causing-weight-gain/

Flay, B. (n.d.). *Layered Smoothies*. Food Network.
https://www.foodnetwork.com/recipes/bobby-flay/layered-smoothies-recipe-2113028

Food Network. (n.d.). *Frozen Fruit Smoothies*. Food Network.
https://www.foodnetwork.com/recipes/food-network-kitchen/frozen-fruit-smoothies-recipe-1914927#/

Funke, L. (2013a, June 18). *Peanut Butter and Jelly Protein Smoothie*. Fit Foodie Finds.
https://fitfoodiefinds.com/peanut-butter-and-jelly-protein-smoothie/

Funke, L. (2013b, December 30). *Dark Chocolate Peppermint Protein Shake*. Fit Foodie Finds.
https://fitfoodiefinds.com/dark-chocolate-peppermint-protein-shake/

Funke, L. (2019, October 4). *Strawberry Protein Shake (5 ingredients!)*. Fit Foodie Finds.
https://fitfoodiefinds.com/strawberry-cheesecake-protein-smoothie/

Funke, L. (2020, January 5). *Best Protein Shakes (30+ flavors!)*. Fit Foodie Finds.
https://fitfoodiefinds.com/best-protein-shakes/

Gemmell, S. (n.d.). *Are frozen berry smoothies good for me?* Super Cubes.
https://supercubes.com.au/blogs/cubes/are-frozen-berry-smoothies-good-for-me

Gudzune, K. A., Doshi, R. S., Mehta, A. K., Chaudhry, Z. W., Jacobs, D. K., Vakil, R. M., …
Clark, J. M. (2015). Efficacy of Commercial Weight-Loss Programs. *Annals of Internal Medicine*, *162*(7), 501. https://doi.org/10.7326/m14-2238

Gunnars, K. (2018a, June 29). *10 Health Benefits of Kale*. Healthline.
https://www.healthline.com/nutrition/10-proven-benefits-of-kale#TOC_TITLE_HDR_9

Gunnars, K. (2018b, June 29). *12 Proven Health Benefits of Avocado*. Healthline.
https://www.healthline.com/nutrition/12-proven-benefits-of-avocado#TOC_TITLE_HDR_3

Hasselbrink, K. (2013a, December 28). *Banana Almond Smoothie*. Bon Appétit.
https://www.bonappetit.com/recipe/banana-almond-smoothie

Hasselbrink, K. (2013b, December 30). *Avocado Smoothie*. Bon Appétit.
https://www.bonappetit.com/recipe/avocado-smoothie-2

Hill, A. (2018, November 28). *10 Surprising Benefits of Honeydew Melon*. Healthline.
https://www.healthline.com/nutrition/honeydew#TOC_TITLE_HDR_7

Hill, A. (2020, May 11). *Are Smoothies Good for You?* Healthline.
https://www.healthline.com/nutrition/are-smoothies-good-for-you#benefits

Hughes, C. (2019, April 9). *Immune Boosting Smoothie*. Heart Fully Nourished.
https://heartfullynourished.com/elderberry-immune-boosting-smoothie/

Jennings, K.-A. (2017, May 31). *5 Impressive Health Benefits of Acai Berries*. Healthline.
https://www.healthline.com/nutrition/benefits-of-acai-berries#TOC_TITLE_HDR_7

K, A. (2013, June 7). *Blueberry & Peanut Butter Green Smoothie*. Amanda k. by the Bay.
http://amandakbythebay.blogspot.com/2013/06/blueberry-peanut-butter-green-smoothie.html

Killoran, E. (n.d.). *Are Smoothies Healthy? Are They Good for Weight Loss? | Pritikin Diet*.
Pritikin. https://www.pritikin.com/are-smoothies-healthy-weight-loss

Kitchen Treaty. (2016, January 9). *Mango-Coconut Green Smoothie*. Kitchen Treaty.
https://www.kitchentreaty.com/vegan-mango-coconut-green-smoothie/

Kubala, J. (2018, February 26). *7 Benefits and Uses of CBD Oil (Plus Side Effects)*. Healthline.
https://www.healthline.com/nutrition/cbd-oil-benefits#TOC_TITLE_HDR_5

Leech, J. (2018a, September 6). *9 Evidence-Based Health Benefits of Almonds*. Healthline.
https://www.healthline.com/nutrition/9-proven-benefits-of-
almonds#TOC_TITLE_HDR_6

Leech, J. (2018b, October 9). *10 Proven Health Benefits of Blueberries*. Healthline.
https://www.healthline.com/nutrition/10-proven-benefits-of-
blueberries#TOC_TITLE_HDR_5

Leone, B. (2017, February 9). *Acai Power House Bowl*. Bon Appétit.
https://www.bonappetit.com/recipe/acai-power-house-bowl

Link, R. (2020, February 25). *7 Proven Ways Matcha Tea Improves Your Health*. Healthline.
https://www.healthline.com/nutrition/7-benefits-of-matcha-tea#3.-Boosts-brain-function

Mandl, E. (2018, March 8). *Elderberry: Benefits and Dangers*. Healthline.
https://www.healthline.com/nutrition/elderberry#health-benefits

Marx Foods. (2010, June 14). *Huckleberry Smoothie*. Marx Foods Blog.
https://marxfood.com/huckleberry-smoothie-recipe/

McKeown, S. (2020, June 22). *6 Superfood Smoothies to Clear Your Skin and Make It Glow*.
ZELEN Life. https://zelenlife.com/smoothies-clear-skin/

McMichael, C. (2018, April 16). *Healthy Mango Banana Smoothie*. Jar Of Lemons.
https://www.jaroflemons.com/healthy-mango-banana-smoothie/

McMichael, C. (2020, March 16). *The BEST Tropical Smoothie Recipe*. Jar Of Lemons.
https://www.jaroflemons.com/tropical-breakfast-smoothie/

Mills, J. (2017, February 5). *10 Reasons to Eat Huckleberries*. Healthy Builderz.
www.healthybuilderz.com. https://www.healthybuilderz.com/10-reasons-eat-
huckleberries/

Mind-Body-Vision. (2015, July 14). *Birthday Cake Protein Shake {Healthy, Dairy-Free, Paleo}*.
MIND-BODY-VISION. http://kelleyandcricket.com/birthday-cake-protein-shake/

Morocco, C. (2018, May 22). *Blueberry, Lime, and Cashew Smoothies*. Bon Appétit.
https://www.bonappetit.com/recipe/blueberry-lime-and-cashew-smoothies

Morris, R. (2014, October 16). *6 Health Benefits of Black Currant*. Healthline.
https://www.healthline.com/health/health-benefits-black-currant#boosts-immune-system

National Center for Complementary and Integrative Health. (2019, September). *"Detoxes" and
"Cleanses": What You Need To Know*. National Center for Complementary and
Integrative Health. https://www.nccih.nih.gov/health/detoxes-and-cleanses-what-you-
need-to-know

Nourish. (n.d.). *Green Smoothies: Are They Good for You?* WebMD.
https://www.webmd.com/diet/green-smoothies-are-they-good-for-you#1

Pathak, N. (2020, September 21). *Health Benefits of Cranberries*. WebMD. https://www.webmd.com/food-recipes/health-benefits-cranberries

Petre, A. (2020, June 10). *Are Cashews Good for You? Nutrition, Benefits, and Downsides*. Healthline. https://www.healthline.com/nutrition/are-cashews-good-for-you#type-2-diabetes

Platings and Pairings. (2020, March 11). *Healthy Blackberry Smoothie*. Platings + Pairings. https://www.platingsandpairings.com/blackberry-smoothie-recipe-no-banana/#wprm-recipe-container-22725

Pretty Little Apron. (2014, December 6). *Strawberry Pomegranate Green Smoothie*. Pretty Little Apron. http://www.3boysunprocessed.com/strawberry-pomegranate-green-smoothie/

Rabbit Food for my Bunny Teeth. (2014, February 10). *Snickerdoodle Green Smoothie*. Rabbit Food For My Bunny Teeth. https://rabbitfoodformybunnyteeth.com/snickerdoodle-green-smoothie/

Ray, R. (n.d.). *Frothy-Chilly Fruit Smoothies*. Food Network. https://www.foodnetwork.com/recipes/rachael-ray/frothy-chilly-fruit-smoothies-recipe-1915796#/

Richter, E. (2019a, March 30). *Healthy Banana Protein Shake*. Fit Foodie Finds. https://fitfoodiefinds.com/healthy-banana-shake/

Richter, E. (2019b, April 11). *Superfood Protein Smoothie*. Fit Foodie Finds. https://fitfoodiefinds.com/superfood-protein-smoothie/

Richter, E. (2019c, April 12). *Dark Chocolate Protein Date Smoothie*. Fit Foodie Finds. https://fitfoodiefinds.com/dark-chocolate-date-protein-smoothie/

Rogers, P., & Shahrokni, R. (2018). A Comparison of the Satiety Effects of a Fruit Smoothie, Its Fresh Fruit Equivalent and Other Drinks. *Nutrients*, *10*(4), 431. https://doi.org/10.3390/nu10040431

Saffitz, C. (2015a, December 15). *Tropical Carrot, Ginger, and Turmeric Smoothie*. Bon Appétit. https://www.bonappetit.com/recipe/tropical-carrot-ginger-and-turmeric-smoothie

Saffitz, C. (2015b, December 16). *Berry, Beet, Mint, Lime, and Chia Seed Smoothie*. Bon Appétit. https://www.bonappetit.com/recipe/berry-beet-mint-lime-chia-seed-smoothie

Schroder, J. M. (2019). Seeing is believing: Vitamin A promotes skin health through a host-derived antibiotic. *Cell Host & Microbe*, *25*(6), 777–788. https://doi.org/10.1016/j.chom.2019.05.011

Shoemaker, S. (2019, July 3). *9 Surprising Benefits of Tahini*. Healthline. https://www.healthline.com/nutrition/tahini-benefits#TOC_TITLE_HDR_7

Shubrook, N. (n.d.). *The health benefits of blackberries*. BBC Good Food. https://www.bbcgoodfood.com/howto/guide/health-benefits-blackberries#:~:text=Blackberries%20contain%20a%20wide%20array

Slajerova, M. (2014, July 24). *Low-Carb Summer Blackcurrant Smoothie*. KetoDiet. https://ketodietapp.com/Blog/lchf/Summer-Blackcurrant-Smoothie

Stockton, L. (2020, June 30). *How to Keep Your Produce Fresh for Weeks (Hint: It's Not Always in the Fridge)*. Wirecutter: Reviews for the Real World. https://www.nytimes.com/wirecutter/blog/keep-your-produce-fresh/

Styles at Life. (2019, September 17). *14 Best Boysenberry Benefits + Nutrition Facts & Side Effects*. Styles At Life. https://stylesatlife.com/articles/boysenberries-benefits/

Sunshine, A. (2013, March 21). *Tropical Green Smoothie (The BEST Green Smoothie!)*. Averie Cooks. https://www.averiecooks.com/tropical-green-smoothie/

Tan, K. W., Graf, B. A., Metra, S. R., & Stephan, I. D. (2015). Daily consumption of a fruit and vegetable smoothie alters facial skin color. *Plos One*, *10*(7). https://doi.org/10.1371/journal.pone.0133445

The Blendery. (2020, December 22). *Are Smoothies Good For Weight Loss? Here's What The Science Says...*The Blendery. https://www.theblendery.com/weight-loss-smoothies/

Walsh, K. (2015, December 15). *How to Make a Smoothie Better (and Cheaper) Than Any You Can Buy*. Better Homes & Gardens. https://www.bhg.com/recipes/breakfast/smoothies/how-to-make-a-smoothie/

WebMD. (n.d.). *Boysenberry-Banana Blast*. WebMD. https://www.webmd.com/food-recipes/boysenberry-banana-blast